Edwardian Ladies' Hat Fashions

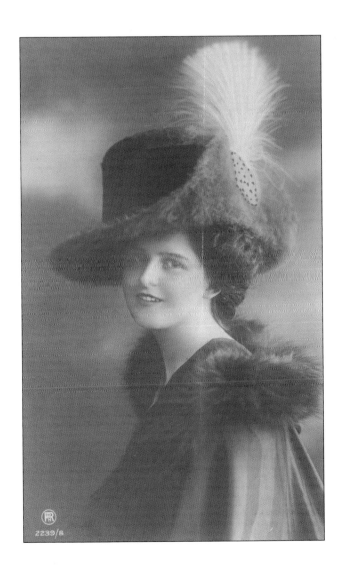

2239/8

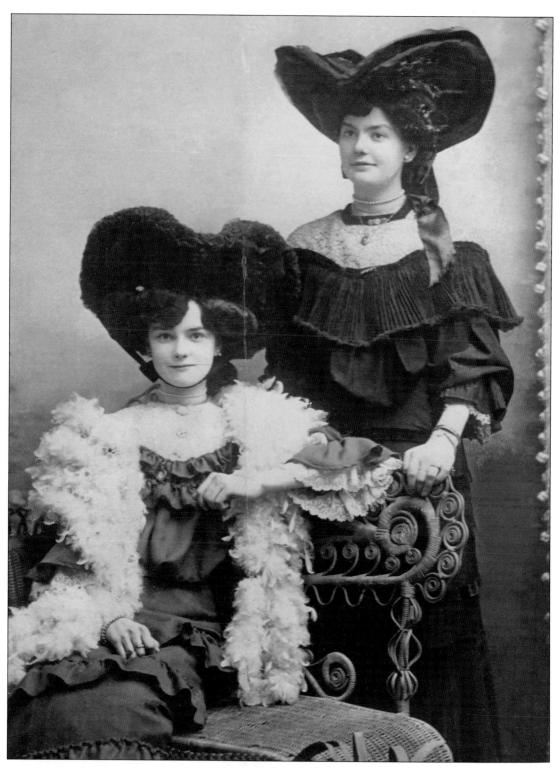

Keeping it in the family – the author's own grandmother 'Nana Rosie' (foreground) and her sister great aunt Maud taken in around 1910. An attractive young pair, all got up in their giant hats, frills and a boa. Love you girls.

Edwardian Ladies' Hat Fashions

'Where Did You Get That Hat?'

AN ILLUSTRATED HISTORY OF
EDWARDIAN LADIES' HATS AND
THE FEATHER INDUSTRY OF THE PERIOD

Peter Kimpton

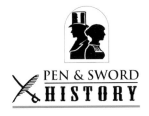

PEN & SWORD
HISTORY

First published in Great Britain in 2017 by
PEN AND SWORD HISTORY
an imprint of
Pen and Sword Books Ltd
47 Church Street
Barnsley
South Yorkshire S70 2AS

ISBN 978 1 47388 129 7

Printed and bound by Replika Press Pvt. Ltd, India

Typeset in Gill Sans by Chic Graphics, UK

Pen & Sword Books Ltd incorporates the imprints of
Pen & Sword Archaeology, Atlas, Aviation, Battleground, Discovery,
Family History, History, Maritime, Military, Naval, Politics, Railways,
Select, Social History, Transport, True Crime,
Claymore Press, Frontline Books, Leo Cooper, Praetorian Press,
Remember When, Seaforth Publishing and Wharncliffe.

For a complete list of Pen and Sword titles please contact
Pen and Sword Books Limited
47 Church Street, Barnsley, South Yorkshire, S70 2AS, England
E-mail: enquiries@pen-and-sword.co.uk
Website: www.pen-and-sword.co.uk

Contents

Dedication

To my beloved Rose, my ever bright and shining star. For your love, your loyalty and happy smile, your valued critiques and totally unstinting patience in trying to help me master my computer and for your stoicism in failure!

And for dearest Jess – one of life's special people – an ordinary yet outstanding and joyous human being who left us in 2005 in her nineties. Born in 1912 – and from an age long since passed, she was an object lesson to us all with the grace, affection, wit and wisdom she showed in accepting all that life sent her way. Your humility and love will stay with us always Jess – God bless you.

Also for my daughters Rachael and Elizabeth, and grandchildren Sam and Tommy, Josie and Henry, Isaac and Esme – for the future with my love. Special mention also to Paul, Chris and Renate.

And not forgetting Nana Rosie, Brian the soldier and 2nd Lieutenant Norman Herbert Kimpton, who was killed aged 20 at Boesinghe near Ypres, in Flanders, on 14 July 1917.

Finally, I would be remiss if I forgot to mention all my many Edwardian 'girlfriends' featured in this book from within my personal postcard archive, who, although sadly now long gone, have remained captured in time, ghosts of the past – ever-happy and ever-beautiful with their enigmatic and knowing smiles still greeting us from over a hundred years ago. And even though we shall never meet, just a small thank you, ladies, for the pleasure you have given.

Acknowledgements

I am particularly indebted to the following who generously gave their time, advice and expertise in compiling information for this work. My thanks to them all.

To my brother Chris Kimpton, for his excellent photographic skills and advice.

Ruth Battersby Tooke and Lisa Little – Curator and Curatorial Assistant respectively of the Norwich Castle Museum Costume and Textile Study Centre.

My grateful thanks to Orla Fitzpatrick – Irish photo-historian, for her kind permission to use Irish Edwardian wedding images from her archive.

Thanks also to Paul Moorehead, Chairman of the Hat Pin Society of Great Britain. (Now sadly disbanded).

Similarly, I must also give special thanks to Jodi Lenocker, President of The American Hatpin Society and Leslie Woodbury (images) for their special assistance.

For her help with the Coco Chanel images and text, I am indebted to Cécile Goddet-Dirles, Direction du Patrimonie, Chanel – Paris.

For their kind permission to use the Hewitt family photograph, I thank Ron Weibe and the Trustees of the Mo Museum, Sheringham, Norfolk.

Also, to Tommy Heywood-Briggs for the use of his Edwardian Bridges family wedding photograph. To Brian Turner and Martin Loader for their help with the Blackpool tram image and the Witney railway station images respectively.

Matt Jeffrey – Senior Programmes Manager, The National Audubon Society of America.

Olivia Betts – Media and Campaigns Co-ordinator at the The Royal Society for the Protection of Birds, UK, and Martin Fowlie – Communications Manager at BirdLife International.

Anne Bissonnette Phd. Curator of the Clothing and Textile Collection – University of Alberta, Canada.

Hilda Boshoff of the C.P. Nel Museum in Oudtshoorn, Western Cape Province, South Africa who has been wonderfully helpful in making available a number of period images in connection with the feather industry in that country.

Noé Auvélius – Communications Officer for both Leighton House Museum and 18, Stafford Terrace (Linley Sambourne House) – London.

The Imperial War Museum, London.

Special thanks also to Alyce Cornyn-Selby of The Hat Museum, (The National Hat Museum) Portland, Oregon, USA for her generous help and input and similarly to Deborah Burke of The Antique Vintage Dress Gallery of Stamford, Connecticut.

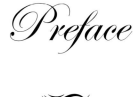

Preface

The Edwardian era was the golden age of millinery, something of a craze one might argue, in which the ornamentation of hats, particularly by the use of exotic feathers, sometimes whole birds and various bits of unfortunate animals, became ever more elaborate. Looking back across the years at how our forebears lived their lives shows, if nothing else, how times, sensitivities, and of course fashions, have changed over the last century or so. In an increasingly technological world it comes, therefore, as something of a surprise to discover today's enormous and growing interest in period fashion around the globe – particularly from the Edwardian era – and it was this interest, in the main, which prompted me to research and write this book.

Today, the modern fashion industries across Europe, the UK and America continue to be amazing innovators, and major employers, which is another sound reason for researching their origins. Having made that point, however, one cannot hide from the fact that in more recent years, the feather, as a fashion accessory, used so widely back in Edwardian times has made something of a 'comeback' via many of the celebrated fashion houses around the globe. Fortunately, these come from environmentally sustainable sources (so we are told) which offers a degree of reassurance in our ever shrinking world – a world in which both animals and birds seem to be forever fighting a rearguard battle and, sadly, losing.

Initially, the basic concept behind this book was to showcase my comprehensive Edwardian postcard archive of beautiful and, at times, almost unreal feather covered female hat fashions of that era and to give the reader a flavour of those early twentieth century years. The work features numerous pretty young ladies of the day from all walks of life and has been purposely written in an unpretentious and non-technical manner. Hopefully you will find the historical background of the Edwardian fashion era and how it related to ladies hat fashions of the period informative. I have also included some amusing happenings and anecdotes here and there in relation to my postcard collecting 'jaunts' over the years in my search for Edwardian ladies and their hats, achieving, I hope, a reader-friendly overview.

However, life is never simple and as I began to research and organise my material for this project, I got something of a nasty surprise as it soon became obvious that there was much more to the subject than I, in my ignorance, had previously imagined.

Little did I realise when viewing my postcards, the carnage that was going on in the background. What had started out in my mind as a fairly light-hearted offering about fashionable, frothy Edwardian ladies' hats based on images from my collection, rapidly turned a very sinister corner. I soon discovered a very brutal and dark story behind all the glamour of the 'Plume Boom' (as it was sometimes known), which was readily depicted on the postcards of the day.

The storm clouds of fashion, aided by the ever-expanding postcard industry, were brewing, and little did unsuspecting bird populations around the world realise what was heading their way! In hindsight, this was an episode in fashion history for which many unthinking, money-seeking individuals of the era, from the northern coasts of Britain, to the Everglades of America and even further afield, should have hung their heads in shame.

Sadly, as you will read further on, making money (and there was much to be made) on the back of incredible cruelty towards birds purely to satisfy ladies' fashions of the day, and the hanging of heads in shame were invariably a considerable distance apart. It really was quite an eye-opener, and not in the best sense of the word at that. Murdering millions of birds just to be able to put their feathers on top of ladies' hats or 'enhance' various fashion accessories doesn't earn the human race many brownie points in my opinion but sadly, extremes often occur when 'crazes' take hold.

Having made that point however, one should emphasise that the ostrich feather industry in South Africa was (and is) a very different scenario; the birds there were usually 'cropped' at regular intervals rather than being cruelly exterminated by the feather hunters. Indeed, to counter accusations of cruelty from around the globe, many feather suppliers and bird breeders were at pains to point out that the feathers they supplied were gathered purely from the birds' natural 'shedding' process. Maybe some were telling the truth?

Over and above this, one has to take into account working conditions and deprivations endured by those at the lower end of the social scale, especially in the millinery sweat shops found in places like New York. Having made these points however, one has to reflect upon the fact that the dreadful goings-on in the early twentieth century, as far as birds were concerned, in a way set the tone for better things to come and the establishment of many great conservation organisations in operation around the world today.

And so read on, but be prepared to be shocked by what was happening in the world of birds and millinery in the early 1900s.

Enter the New Boy

The twentieth century had arrived and the dour and seemingly indestructible Queen Victoria finally departed this world in 1901 – to be reunited with her beloved Albert. Few sovereigns had come to the throne with lower expectations than Edward had, as he saluted the crowd from his splendid black horse at his mother's funeral. The Edwardian era that was to follow, described by some as the 'last hurrah' of Empire, was a distinct, different and certainly very memorable niche in the history of the United Kingdom and, by association, numerous other countries around the world – certainly as far as fashion was concerned. Things were lightening up, although those in high social and fashionable circles can have had little idea of what was going on in the world of birds!

Victoria, who had become something of a recluse after Albert's death, had many times despaired of her eldest son and heir Edward, born in 1841 and known as 'Bertie', for his many indiscretions, wayward behaviour and an undoubted talent for scandalising society. The ageing queen was terrified that he was becoming something of a throwback to the wayward Hanovarians. Indeed, some modern psychologists assess Bertie as having what is known today as Attention Deficit Disorder. In her mind, and indeed others in court circles, the portly boy was significantly lax, had gone off the rails with horse racing, gambling and, of course, the ladies, and was not up to the job of taking over from her. Basically, people did not take him seriously and he was regarded as something of a playboy and philanderer. But having waited nearly sixty years to get to the summit, our man had become somewhat bored with his lot; his nickname of 'Edward the Caresser' was probably pretty well deserved, as the portly Prince commenced upon his historical legacy with (alleged) liaisons with the likes of Jenny Churchill (Winston's mother), Lillie Langtry, and Lady Daisy Brooke – the future Countess of Warwick et al. Some sources at the time put the figure at over fifty known affairs, resulting at one point in the celebrated court case that questioned his involvement with a certain Lady Harriet Mordaunt, and a child (his?) born out of wedlock, which resulted in the unfortunate lady being committed to a lunatic asylum for the rest of her days. But, whatever the truth of the matter, Edward, with the Establishment closing ranks around him, contrived to get away with it.

Across the Channel, Paris – the 'City of Light' – where the citizens had at first been hostile towards Edward, was won over by his charm and in return offered him many 'attractions', including performers such as Sarah Bernhardt and Louise Weber, who used the name *La Goulue* (The Glutton). The city became a great magnet for 'Eddy' as he paid numerous visits to houses of ill repute and particularly the famous brothel – 'Le Chabanais', the well known '*maison de tolerance*'. But looking back, let's not forget that the Parisian courtesans of that era were also great patrons of the fashion world and Edward would have undoubtedly encountered many of them on his visits. The top courtesans had to look good for the class of client whom they sought to attract and for those 'ladies' of easy virtue who had made it to the top so to speak – '*Les Grandes Horizontals*' as they were known – money for fashion was certainly not in short supply. Three of the most famous – '*Les Grandes Trois*' – Emilienne d'Alençon, the very beautiful Liane de Pougy and Caroline Otero (known as La Belle Otero) could, on occasion, be seen in the vicinity of the Bois de Boulogne and other fashionable locations, sporting beautiful, large, feather bedecked hats as they went about their business cementing their social contacts with their clients!

Further east, in affluent Berlin, contemporary film footage shows the city crammed with elegant ladies everywhere, sporting their up to date feathered creations. Whether just strolling the fashionable spots, curtseying before the likes of the Kaiser or Hindenberg at society events, or simply 'being seen' in the many outdoor cafes around such places as the Brandenburg Gate, the fraus and fraulines gave pride of place to their hats. And very elegant they were too.

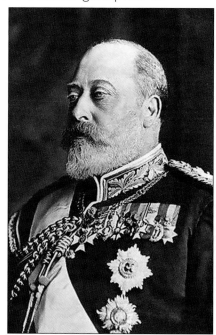

Further east still, the fashion for large hats had even permeated through to the somewhat insulated, though incredibly opulent, court of the Russian royal family. Despite the family's almost convent-like existence, one can often stumble across photographs of Czar Nicholas with his wife Alexandra and their four daughters, Olga, Tatiana, Maria and Anastasia, sporting large feathered hat creations (particularly on one official visit to Romania), at various state or social functions in the years leading up to their murder by the Bolshevics at Yekaterinburg in July 1918.

And yet, back in England, despite all his perceived faults, Edward turned out to be a relatively good king. He had a sort of magical touch – the 'common touch' if you like, and his reign pretty much confounded those who had predicted that he would be a complete disaster. Seen everywhere, Edward was going to do it his way and he loved every minute of it. The new king, a forward-looking man, believed that the Crown should move with the

King Edward VII – the 'Playboy King' and despair of his mother Queen Victoria.

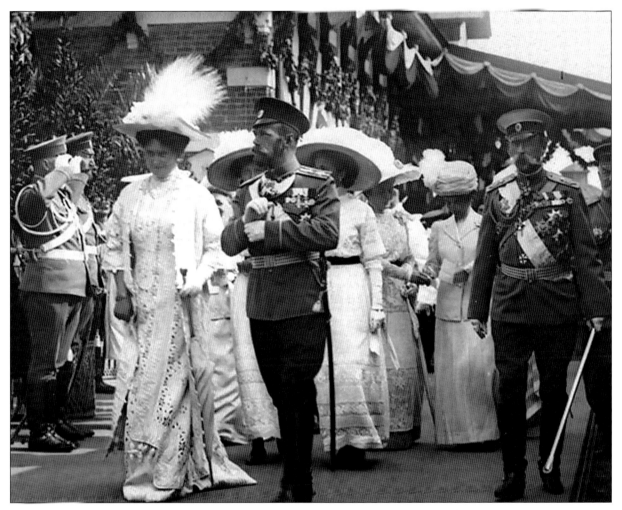

The Russian Czar and his entourage arrive at Borodino railway station in 1912 to celebrate the original 'Battle of Borodino' 100 years earlier. Notice the profusion of large feathered hats on show. *(Image: The Boris Yeltsin Library, St Petersburg, Russia.)*

times. He welcomed anything new, he even learned to ride a bicycle and took up golf, which must have been something of a sight to see. Unsurprisingly, people quickly took to him and he surprised many with his diplomatic skills. He was certainly a sort of 'loose cannon' in today's terms and as we look back, we can see that his accession heralded an era of rapid social change, which somehow contrived to free up what had been a rigid and formal society under his mother's stewardship. Fashion in particular, started to reflect this new-found freedom and creativity, certainly within the realm of ladies' hats, which became increasingly bigger during the first ten years of the twentieth century.

The Edwardian Craze

Although it's now around a hundred or so years since the Edwardian era's craze (and it certainly was a craze) for those enormous and varied ladies' hats, smothered in exotic feathers, and at times whole birds, the interest today – among both young and old – in these stunning creations is bewildering. It is amazing to see the multitude of twenty-first century reproductions on offer from professional manufacturers and talented amateurs around the globe – especially in America. While you will find certain books and an astonishing numbers of reference sources covering a broad spectrum of the history of fashion in general and, to a degree, the feather trade over the last century or so, this particular book focuses on postcards, photographic images and weekly or monthly publications from those niche Victorian and Edwardian periods. Similarly, in the run up to the First World War, hats, hats and more hats, in a bewildering range of designs, in all shapes, sizes and assorted materials, were regarded as the last word – 'le dernier cri' by the ladies of the day.

Although much has been written on the subject, they say a picture is worth a thousand words and, for me, Edwardian fashion – considerably influenced by the Art Nouveau trend – is more vividly brought to life by the evocative images to be found on those postcards of the period. These are not records of earth shattering social events but, in fashion terms, are simply photographic snapshots of what was going on in the daily lives of the ordinary people of the time. Trends come and go, but whatever era you happen to have been born into, fashion, in one form or another, has always held a perennial interest and provided a source of amusement to many of us when we look back at pictures of what we used to wear – thirty, forty, fifty or more years ago. The human race has always been interested in fashion, certainly in modern times and as the writer, H.W.K Collam once put it in his publication *Come Autumn Hand*: 'Nothing is more nostalgic than the modernity of the past'.

The postcards in my own large and diverse collection, garnered over nearly four decades, have somehow survived the last hundred years or so, despite two world wars and many potential disasters along the way – and represent a fashion treasure trove of the period; a pot pourri of pretty girls and 'plumes'. Featuring nearly 1,000 images of young ladies displaying a diverse range of unbelievable accessories, I feel the time is right to share a cross section of my Edwardian 'girlfriends' (and of course their hats).

And such is the enduring attraction of these cards, for me at least, that if one day the 'Postcard Fairy' should suddenly appear and grant me three wishes, I would, without hesitation, travel back in time to those early 1900s with an enormous empty suitcase. There, for mere pennies, I would raid the many street postcard stands and fill my case with all the 'Hats' cards I could get my hands on.

However, fantasies apart and having completed this book, I realised that I still needed a suitable title – maybe something a bit different and appropriate for a book that dedicates itself to the multitude of pretty young things who sported those giant hats that we see in many different scenarios from the early twentieth century. Struggling for a solution, I suddenly remembered from my youth, the late entertainer Stanley Holloway lustily singing the old Victorian music hall song *Where Did You Get That Hat?* composed by Joseph J Sullivan in 1888 (and re-written by James Rolmaz in 1901) and so, with due deference to the composer(s) and thanks to Stanley H and Messrs Sullivan and Rolmaz, I had found my title (or at least part of it).

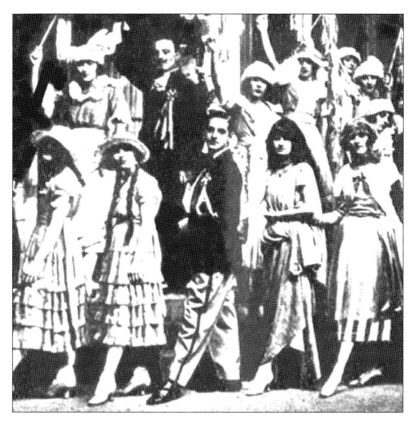

Stanley Holloway's stellar career began in 1910 when he auditioned for *The White Coons*, a concert party variety show. Here he is pictured as René (centre) in *A Night Out* (1920). Amongst his many parts, he famously played Alfred P. Doolittle on Broadway in *My Fair Lady* (1957).

The following pages offer examples of typical hand tinted postcard images from Edwardian times – featuring elegant and beautiful young ladies of the day wearing an amazing range of hats.

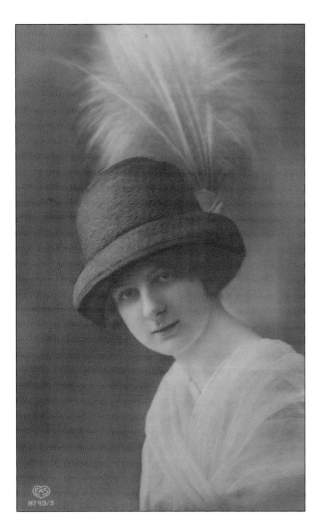

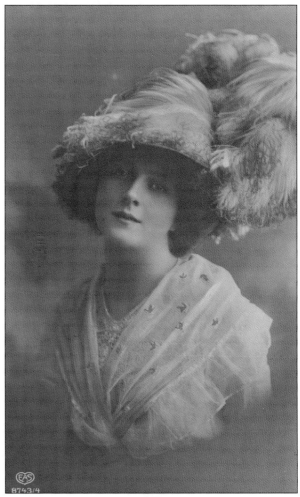

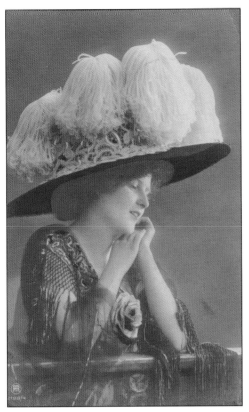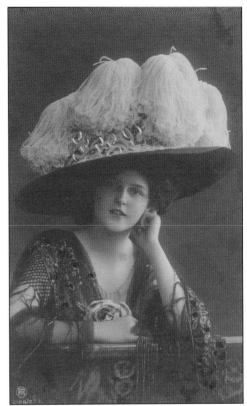
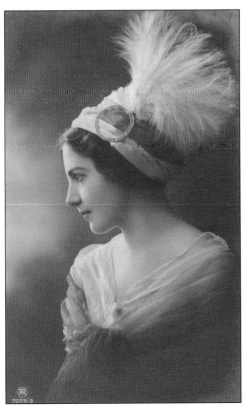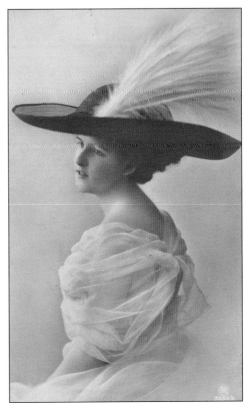

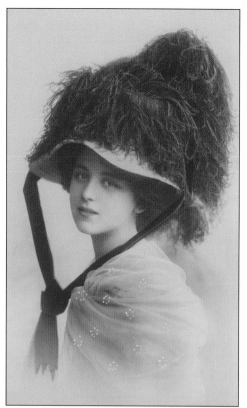
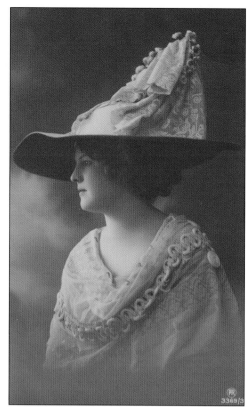
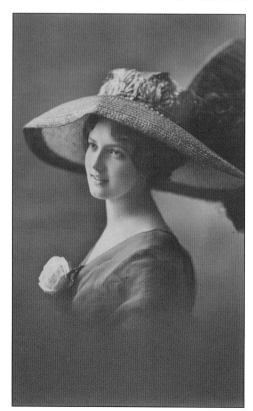
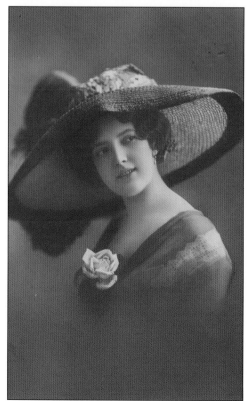

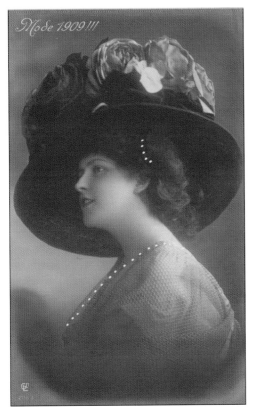

Мода 1909!!!

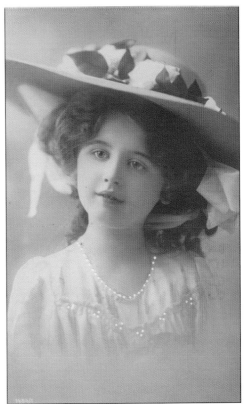

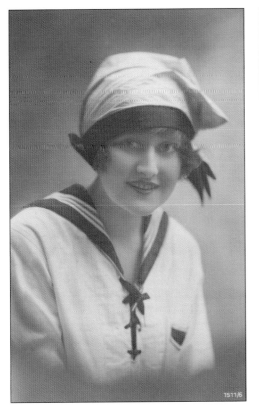

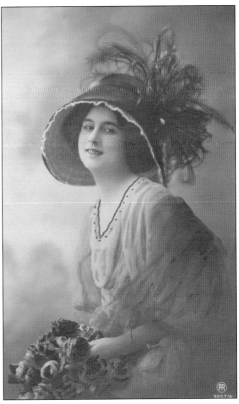

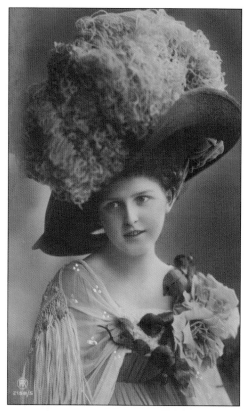

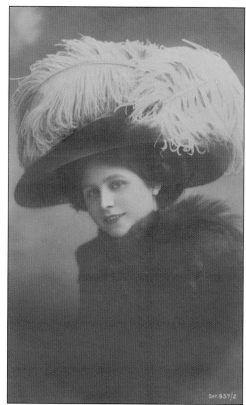

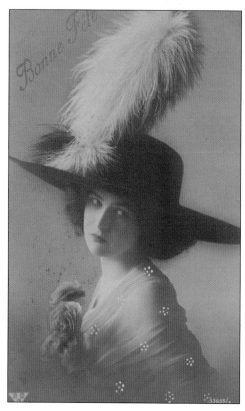

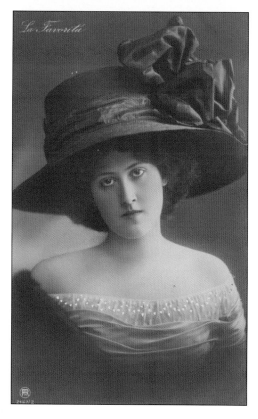

20

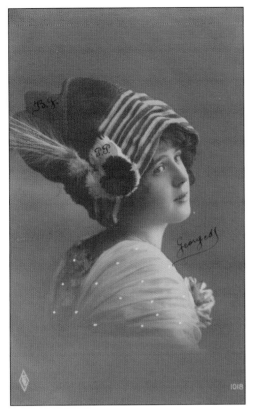

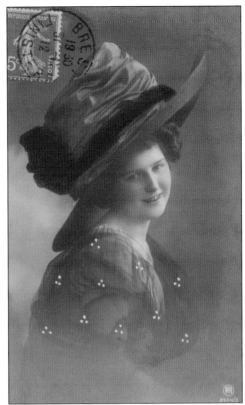

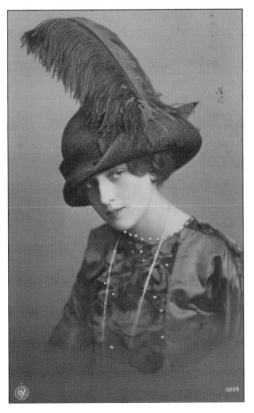

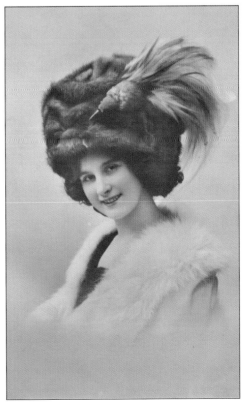

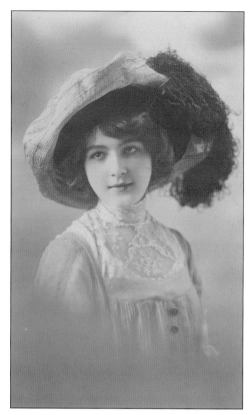
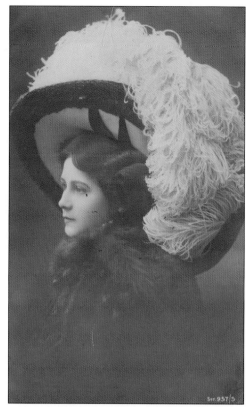
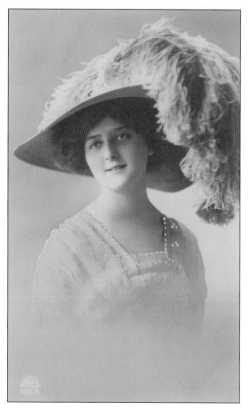
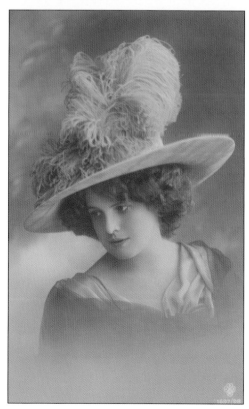

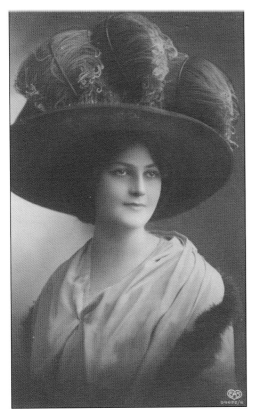
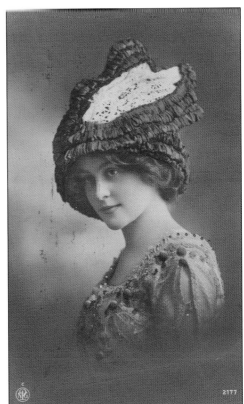
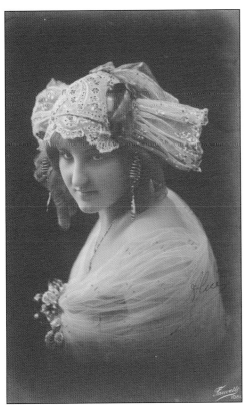
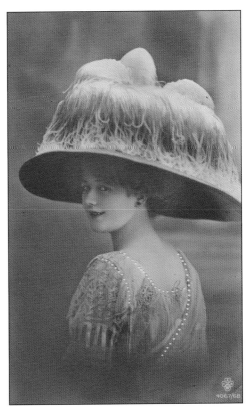

23

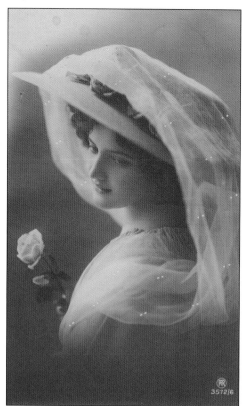

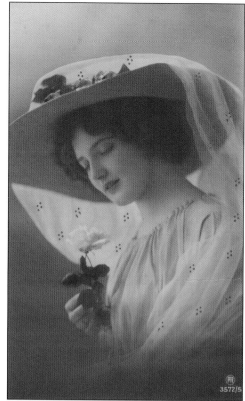

Mode 1909!!!

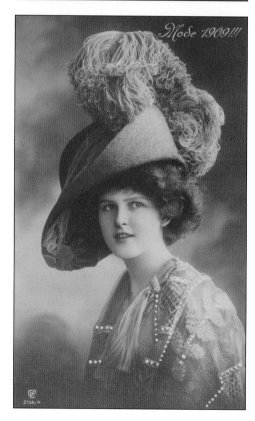

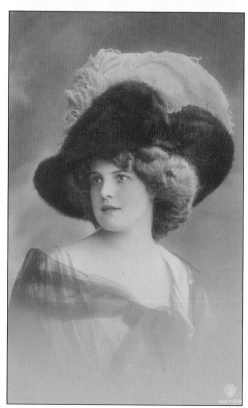

24

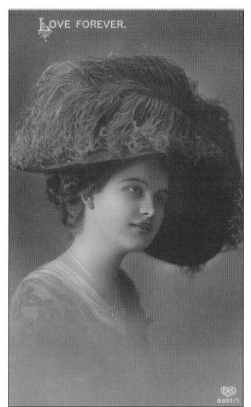

LOVE FOREVER.

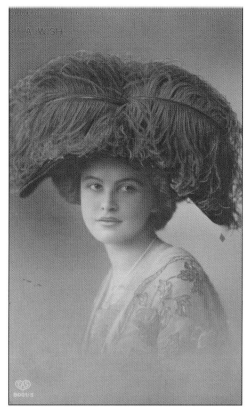

A WISH

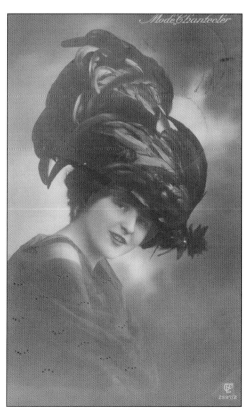

Mode Chantecler

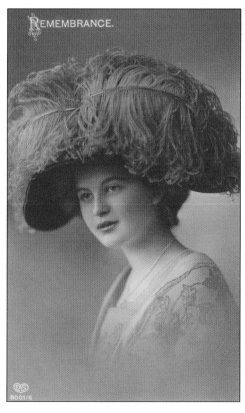

REMEMBRANCE.

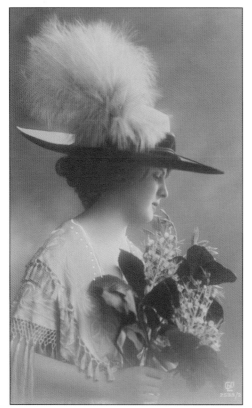

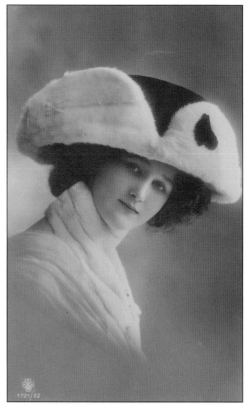

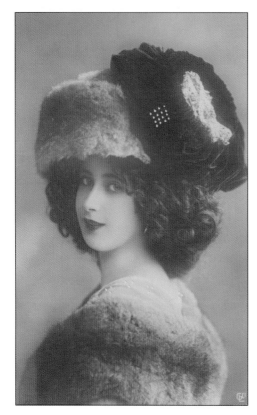

Mode 1909!!!

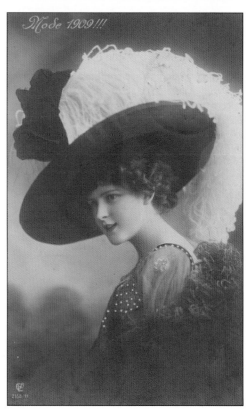

26

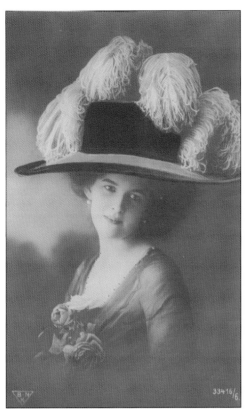
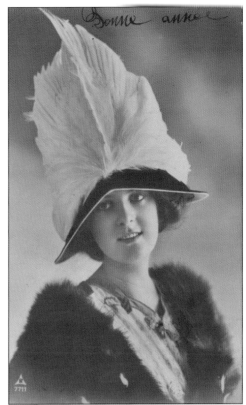
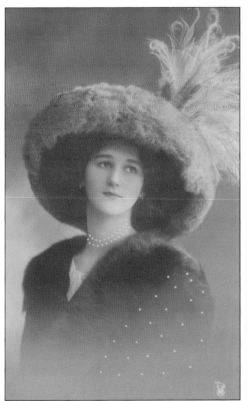
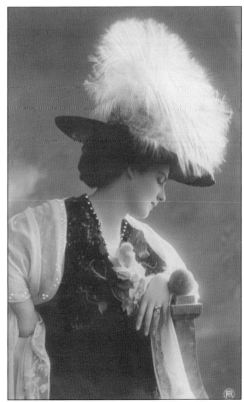

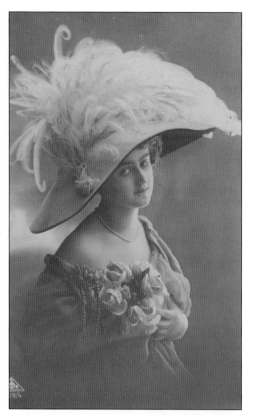
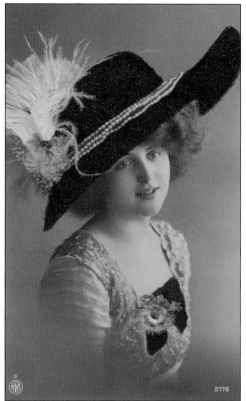
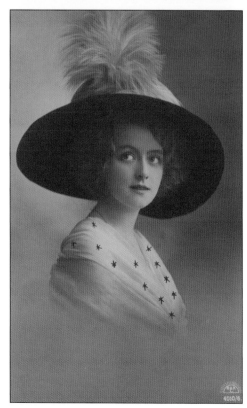
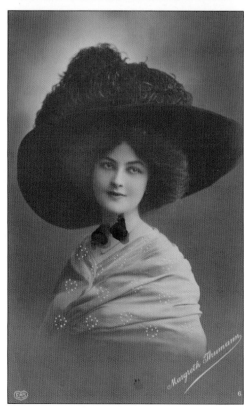

28

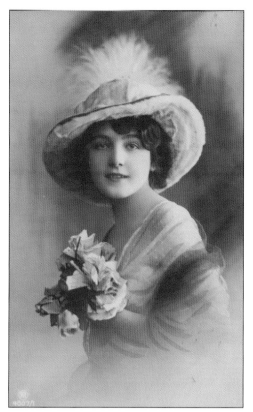

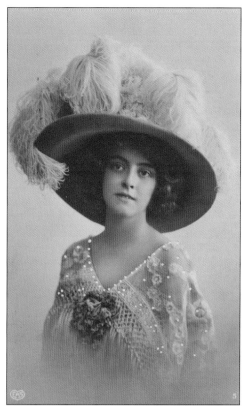

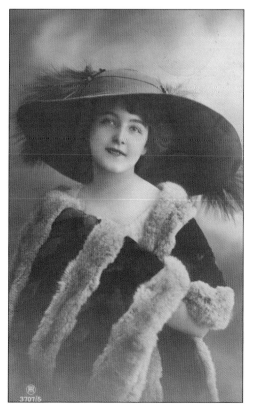

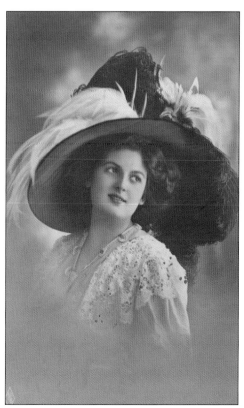

29

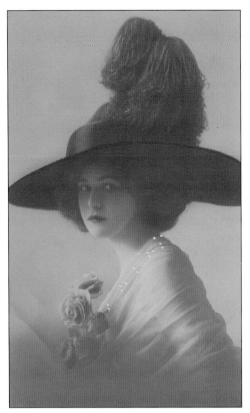

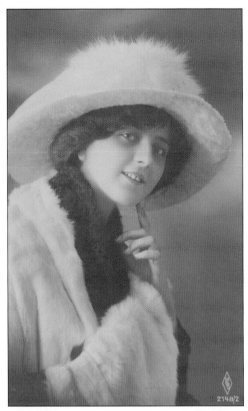

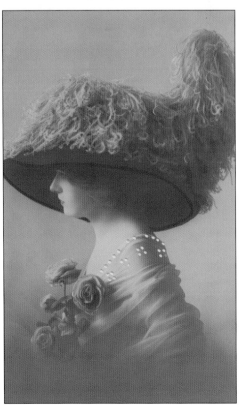

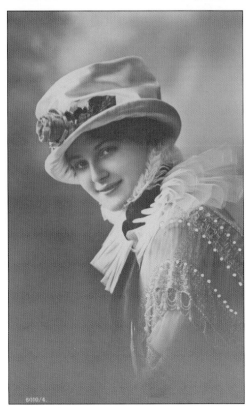

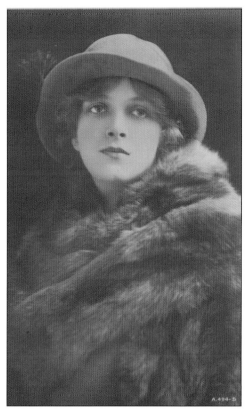

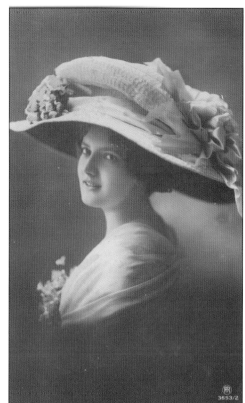

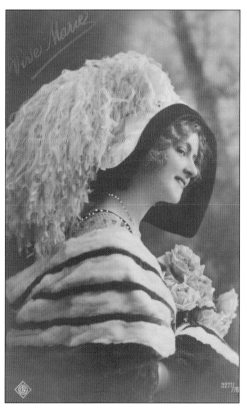

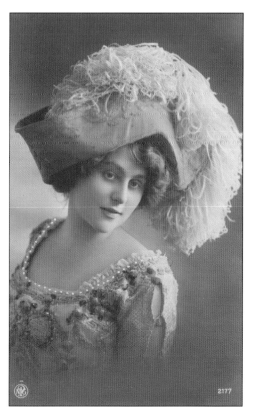

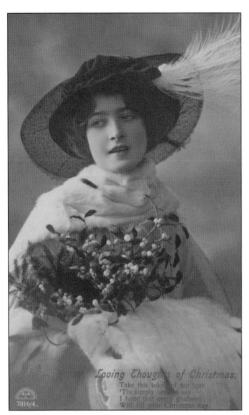

Loving Thoughts of Christmas.
Take this token of my love
'Tis simply meant to try
I hope that every gladness
Will fill your Christmas day

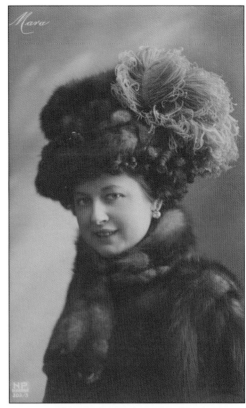

Mara

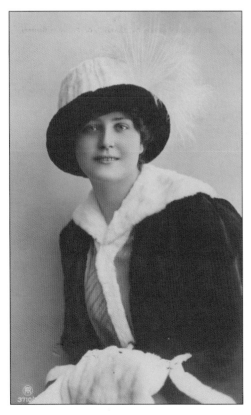

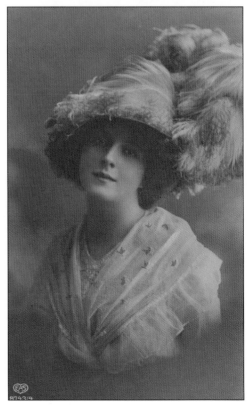

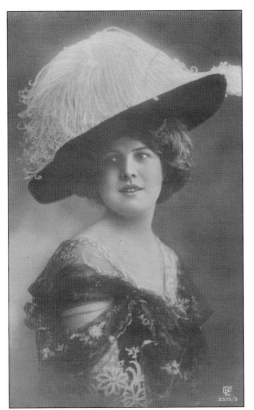
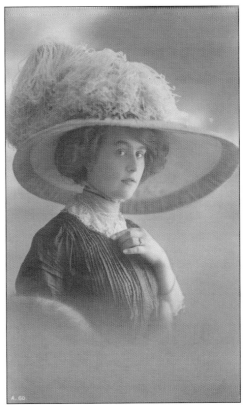
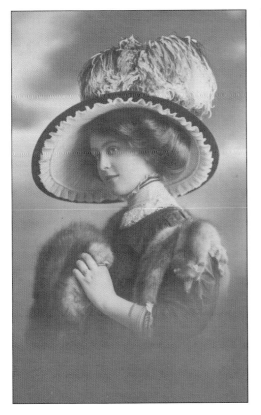
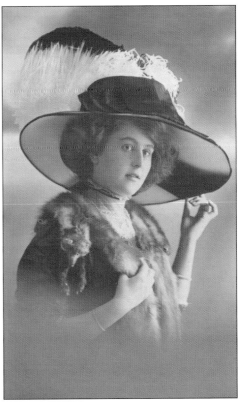

33

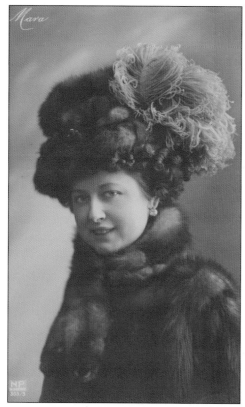
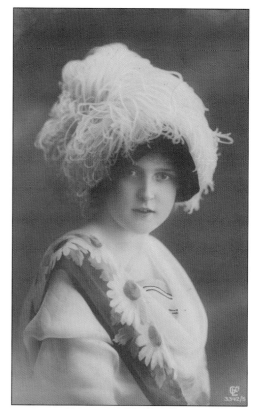
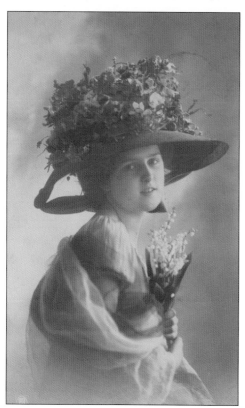
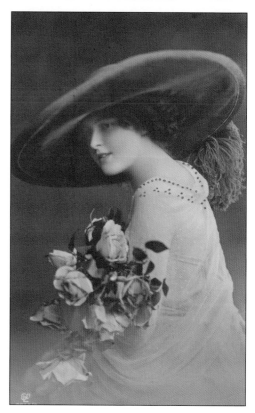

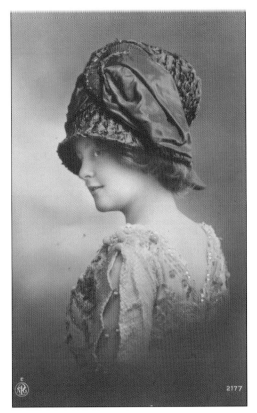
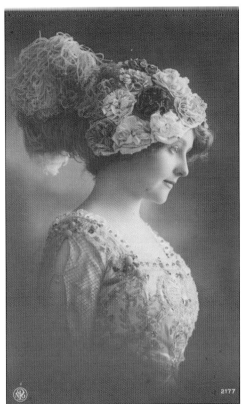
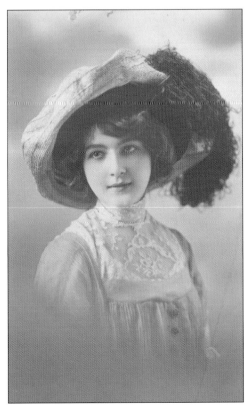
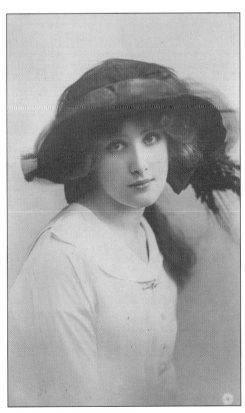

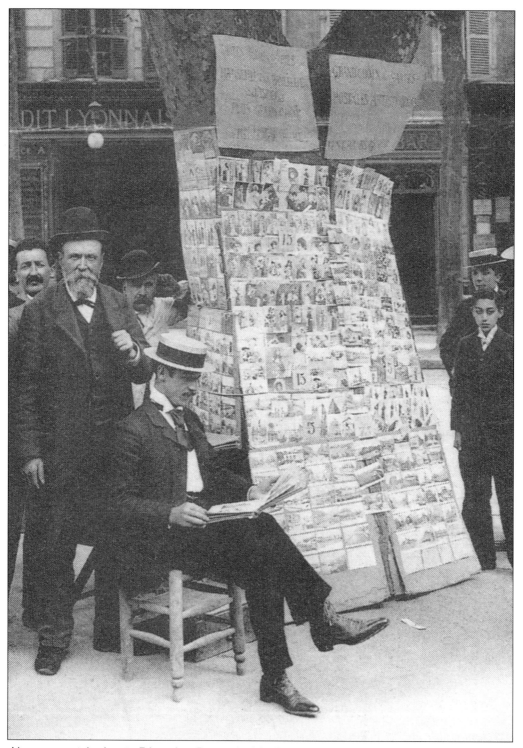

Almost certainly shot in Edwardian Paris, a laid back and snappily dressed street postcard seller, in his straw boater and smart suit, offers a vast range of cards for sale – a number of which feature pretty models displaying ultra sized hats.

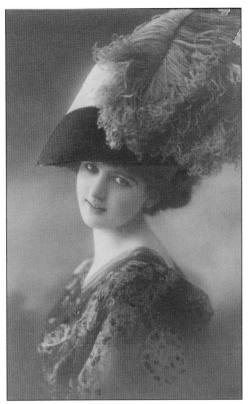
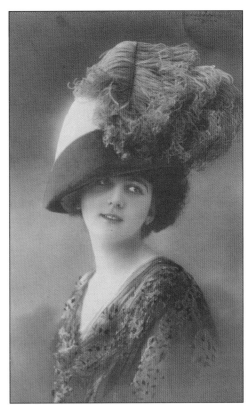
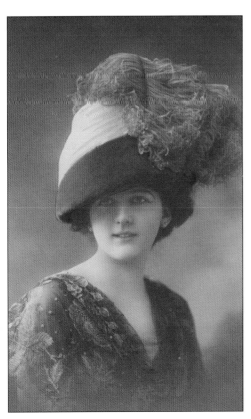
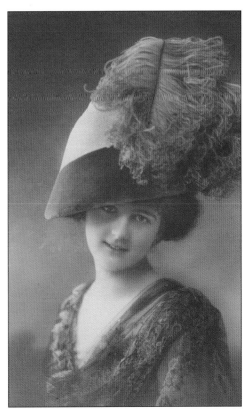

Postcards by the Million

As seasoned postcard collectors (or deltiologists as they are more formally known) will know, there have been thousands of subjects featured on many millions (if not billions) of cards over the years, with the simple messages on the reverse offering, at times, a vivid insight into the world of ordinary folk of the period – the things that surrounded them and the comings and goings that mattered to them in their daily lives. The spectrum is enormous – from trams to theatres, politicians to policemen, and even time spent at the seaside – you name it, it's probably been on a postcard. However, it will come as no surprise that, like so many old things, great numbers of cards have been destroyed over the last century or so by the ravages of the passing years or basic lack of interest. How many wonderful cards have simply finished up in a skip and thence on to landfill? The numbers must be huge. That said, one has to give a belated vote of thanks to all those folk who, however unwittingly, have taken the trouble to keep granny's old family albums and collections of cards tucked away in a drawer or cupboard somewhere, often for decades, and by doing so have fortunately preserved them in decent condition for us to enjoy today.

Thankfully, the vast numbers of cards originally produced means that large quantities have survived into what today has become a huge collecting hobby across the world, offering today's dedicated collector more than an even chance of finding ever more additions to their collections. At postcard fairs around the globe, the supply seems almost endless. There are arguably more postcards around than pretty much anything else in the collecting field and within this massive stock falls the 'Real Photo' or, more commonly, 'Photographic Glamour' cards. In my case, this means young ladies smiling coyly out at us from the early years of twentieth century, wearing an amazing array of headgear including those huge feathered hats or the smaller sized 'Fascinators' as many of them were known then (and still are today), accompanied by furs, stoles (which could often take the form of a whole fox draped around their shoulders), boas and parasols. Maybe, here and there, they can be seen clutching the odd feather fan and a host of frills and fripperies – the sort of thing our grandmothers or great-grandmothers would have worn with relish in their day.

From time to time over the years, my late mother would dig out her collection of old family photographs and we would all have a good laugh at how everybody had changed over time. Since I was a kid, I had always been aware of ladies wearing huge hats by virtue of the fact that amongst those treasured family pictures, we had a charming old photograph – dated around 1910 as it turned out – of my grandmother and her sister (my great aunt Maud) dressed in their best outfits and topped off by a couple of huge hats. (See frontispiece). It seemed almost impossible that my dearest 'Nana Rosie', wrinkled and fragile, busying herself with her knitting, had been the attractive young lady in that picture taken all those years ago. How on earth could this now frail, white-haired old lady once have been this trendy young butterfly?

The following pages feature hats and glamour in profusion – ever more Edwardian postcard images featuring further examples of the astonishing variety of fashionable hats during that period.

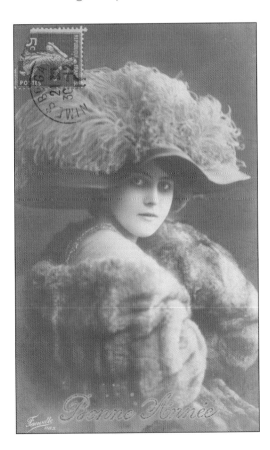
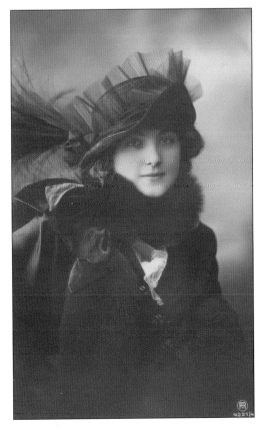

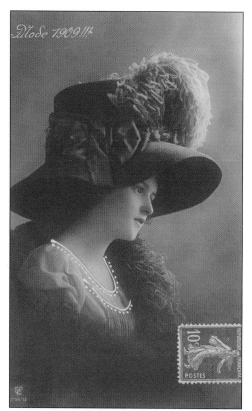

Mode 1909!!!

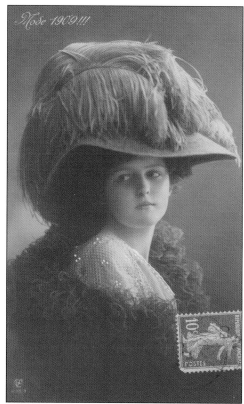

Mode 1909!!!

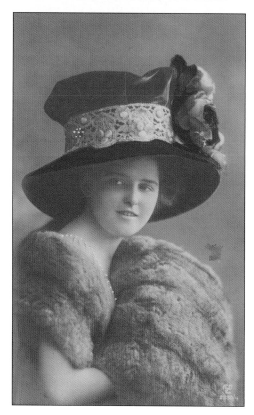

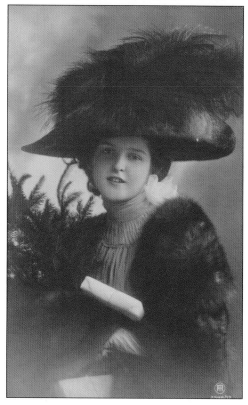

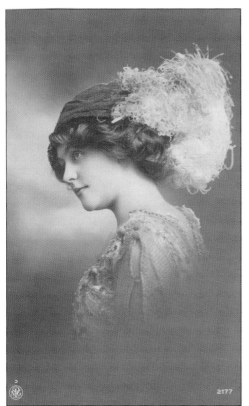

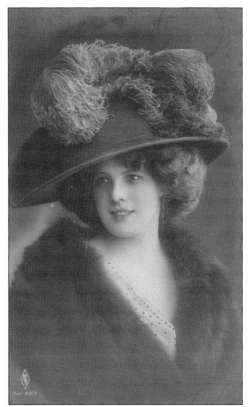

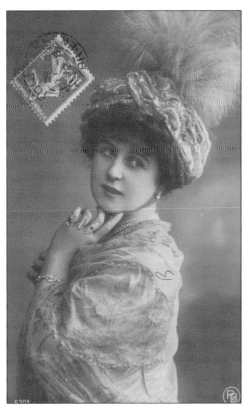

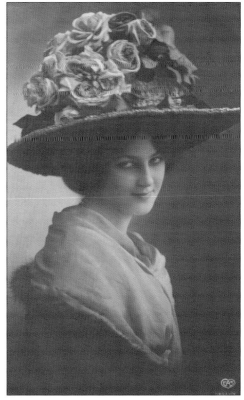

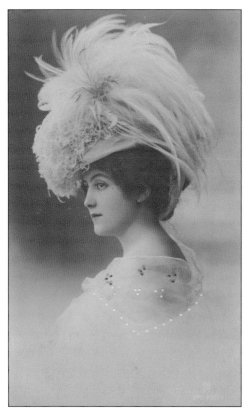

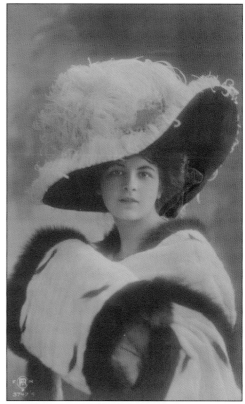

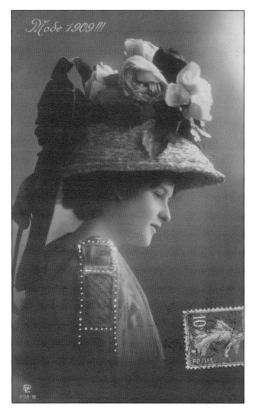

Mode 1909!!!

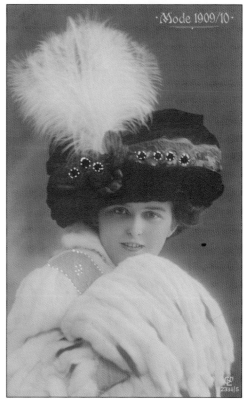

·Mode 1909/10·

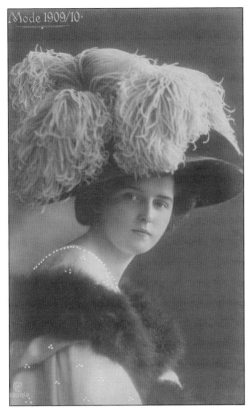

Mode 1909/10

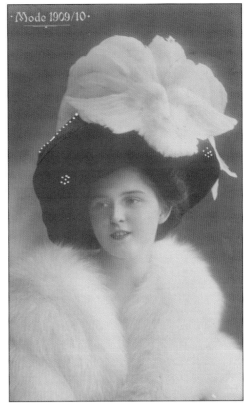

Mode 1909/10

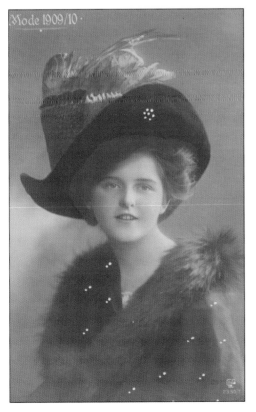

Mode 1909/10

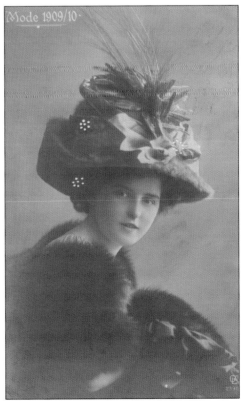

Mode 1909/10

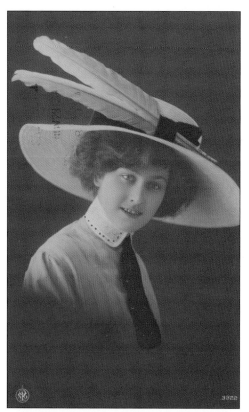
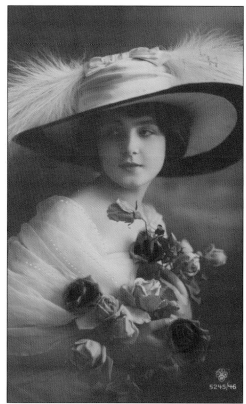
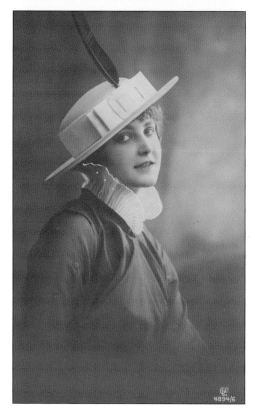
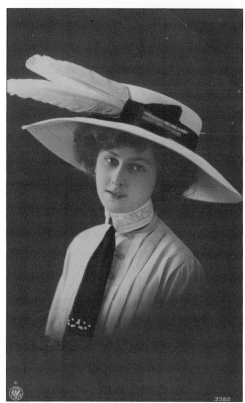

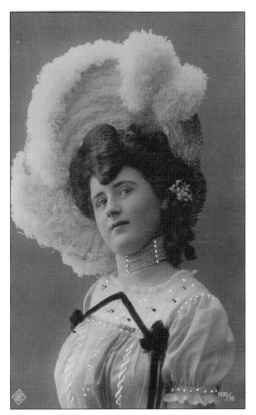

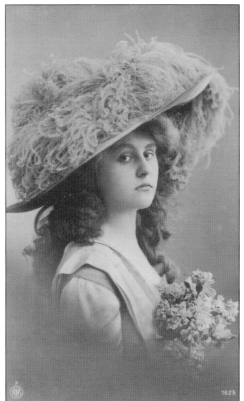

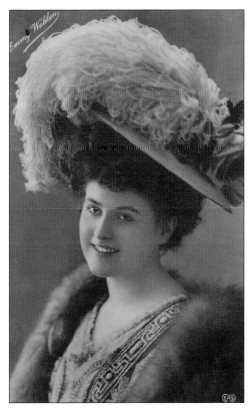

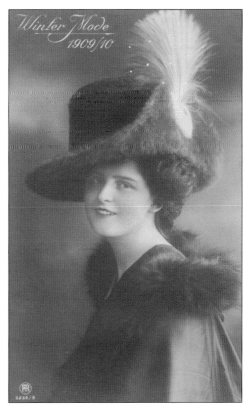

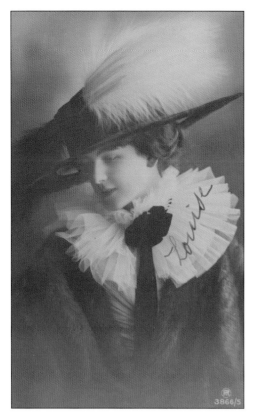 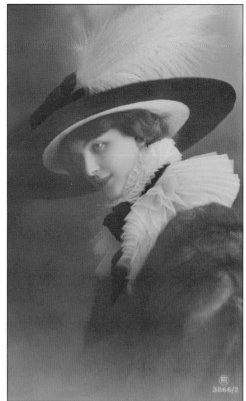

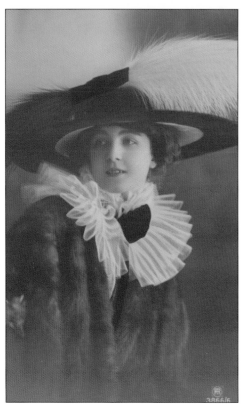 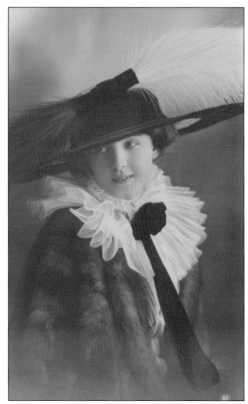

46

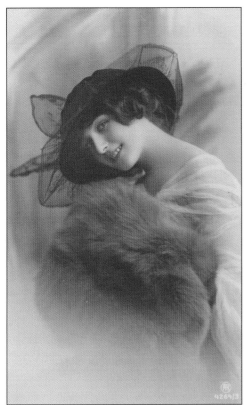
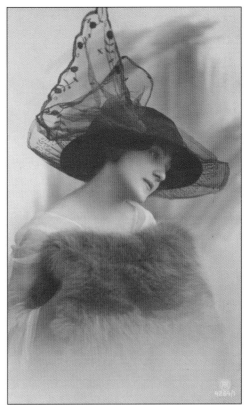
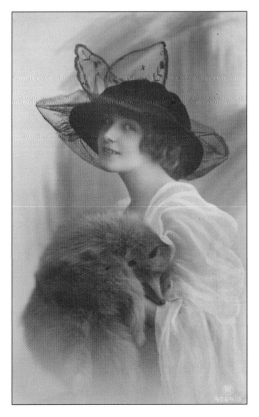
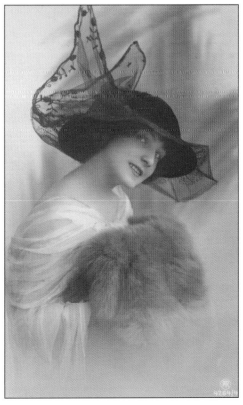

47

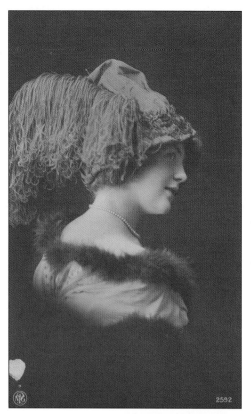
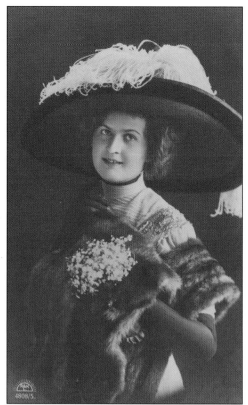
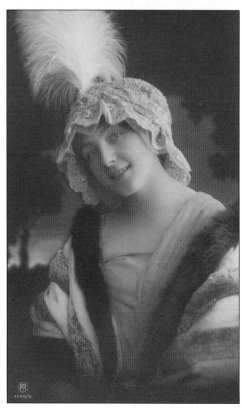
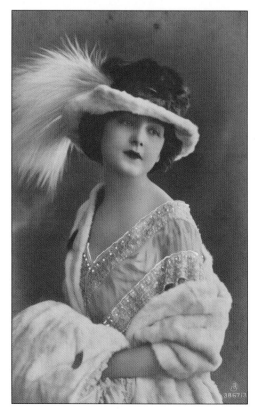

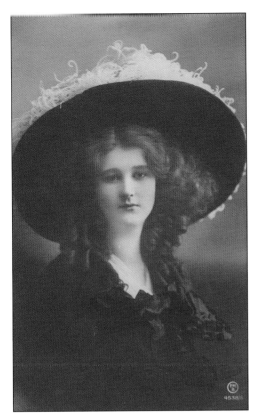
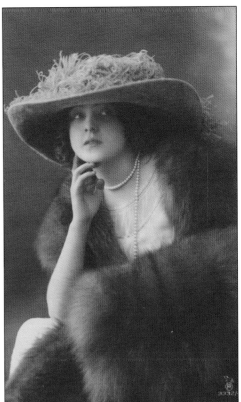
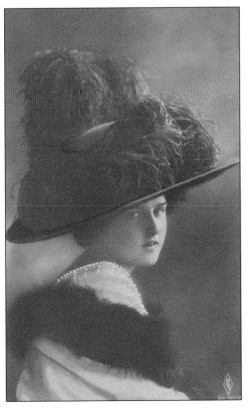
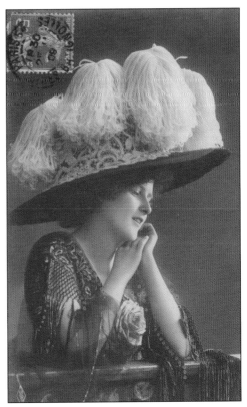

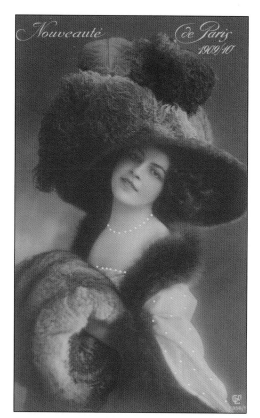

Nouveauté de Paris 1909/10

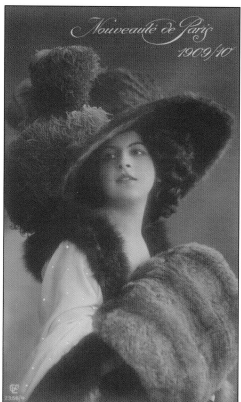

Nouveauté de Paris 1909/10

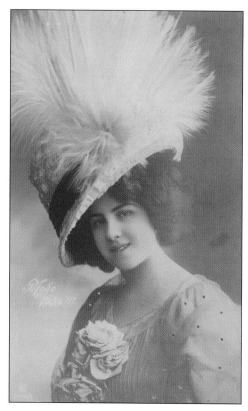

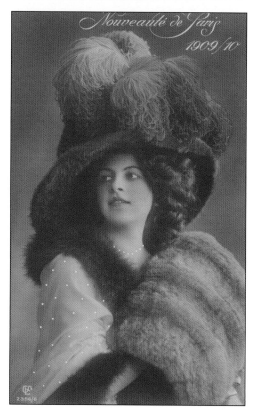

Nouveauté de Paris 1909/10

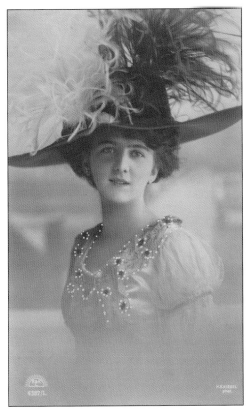

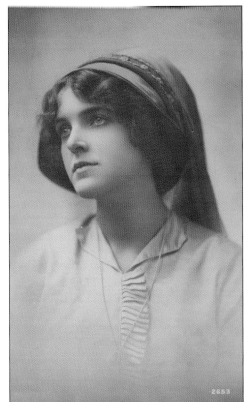

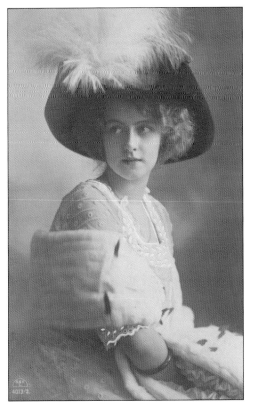

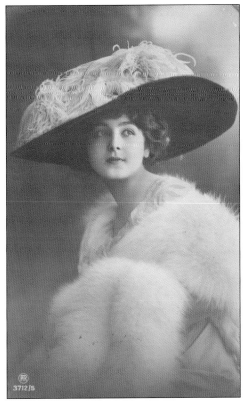

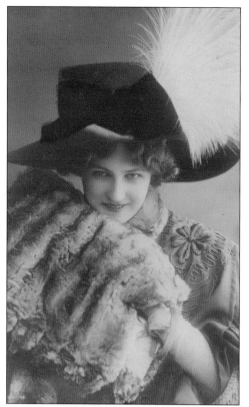

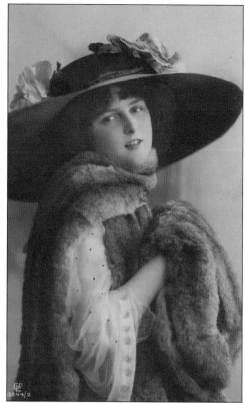

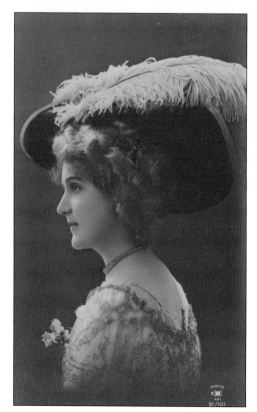

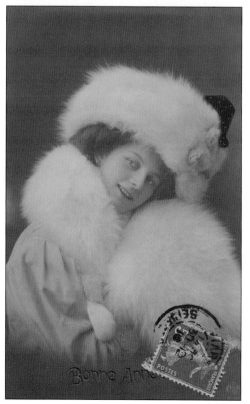

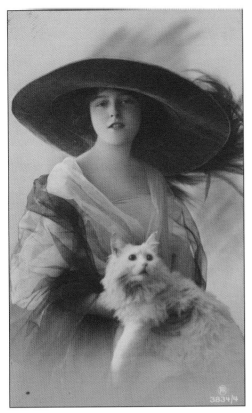

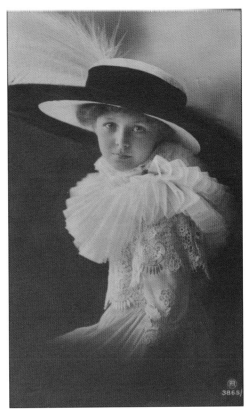

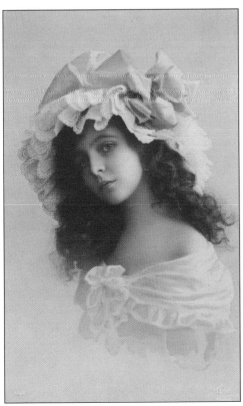

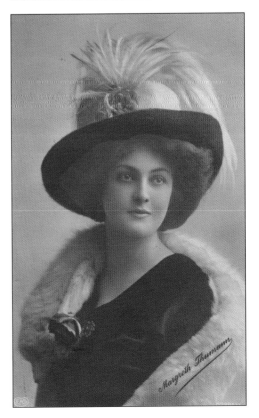

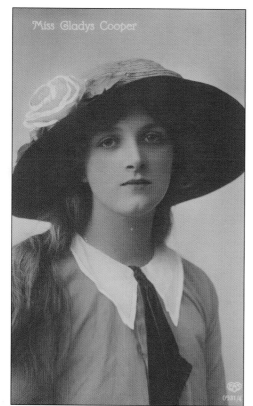

Miss Gladys Cooper

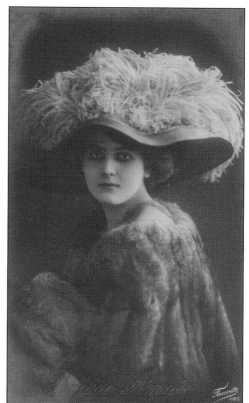

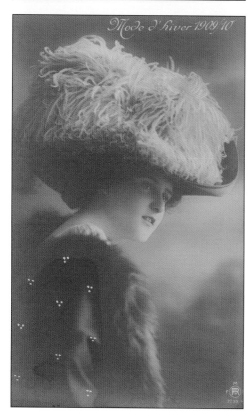

Mode d'hiver 1909/10

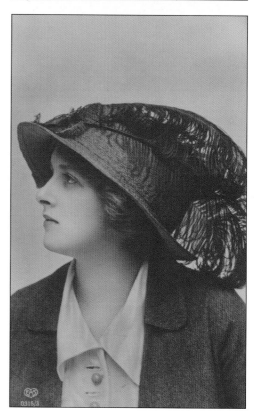

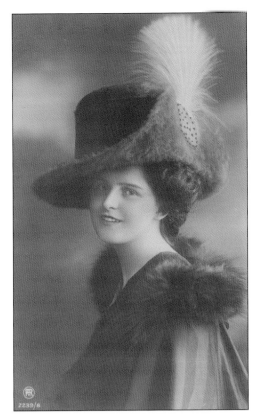
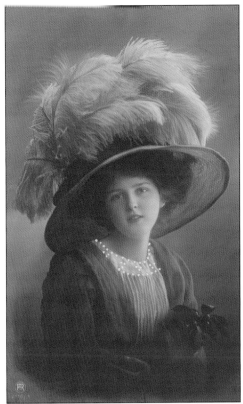
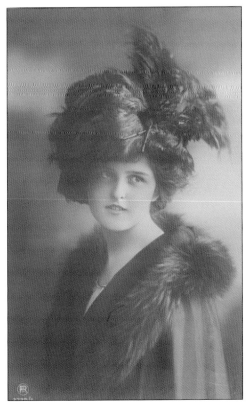
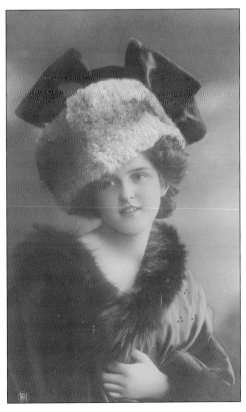

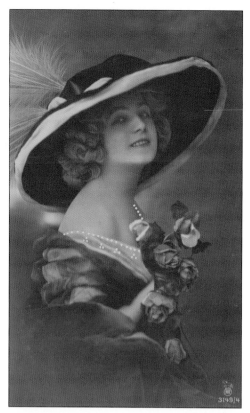
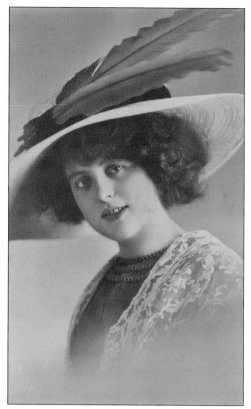
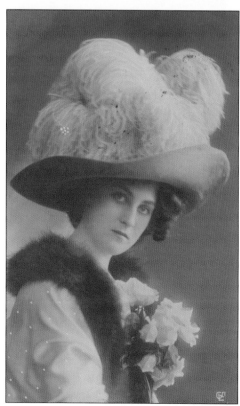
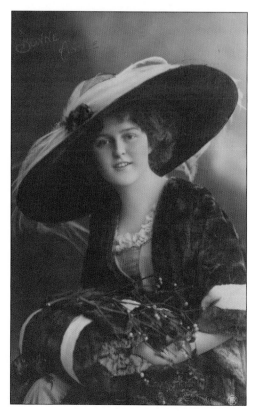

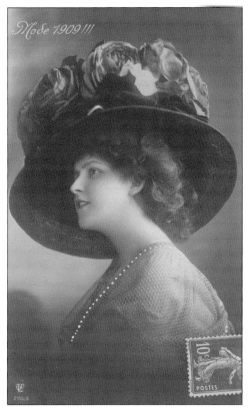

Mode 1909!!!

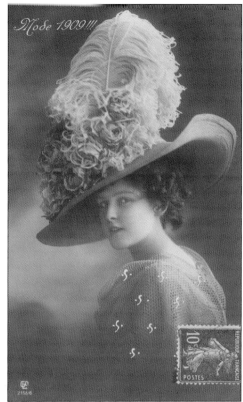

Mode 1909!!!

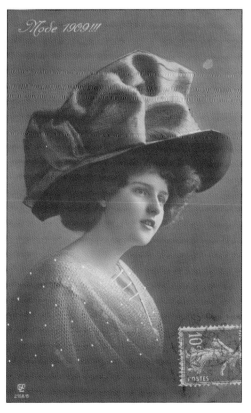

Mode 1909!!!

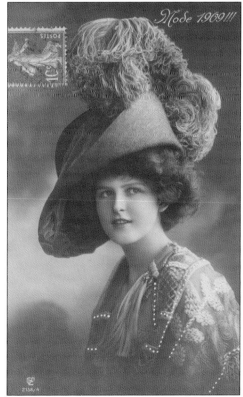

Mode 1909!!!

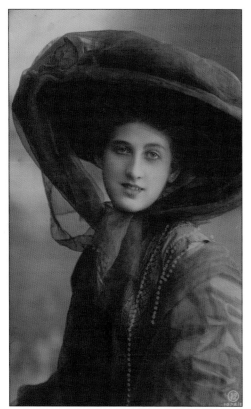
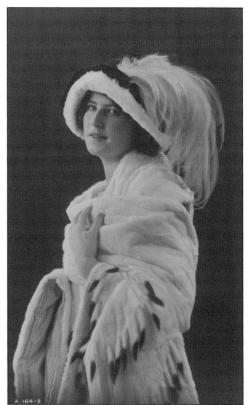
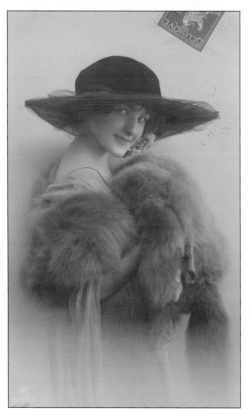
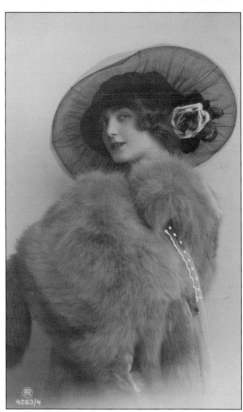

The Merry Widow

Having survived for around those hundred odd years, 'Photographic Glamour' postcards from the Edwardian period have become a rich resource of information and reference for any modern day student of the history of ladies fashion, reflecting a time when the world of couture embarked on one of its periodic flights of fancy – certainly as far as hats and feathers were concerned. A shameful flight some might say.

The popular story is that the age of the big hat, which lasted for around fifteen years (and, as already mentioned, took in the fabulous Art Nouveau period), and ended roughly about the middle of the First World War, came about in part as a result of the fashions that were worn by the actress Lily Elsie, who played the main character of Sonia in Franz Lehar's 1907 stage presentation of *The Merry Widow* (*Die lustige Witwe*) in London. The beautiful Lily, not surprisingly, became one of the Edwardian era's most photographed and well known women, and the trend of 'Merry Widow' hats was eagerly embraced, developed and promoted around the world by the large fashion houses of the day.

In Paris for example, one finds Caroline Reboux (who numbered the Empress Eugénie amongst her clients), in London there was Lucile, the trade name of the well-

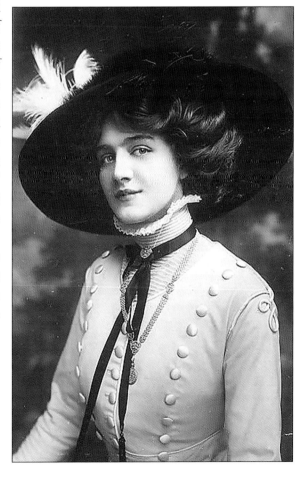

The gorgeous actress – Miss Lily Elsie. Former child star and doyenne of the music hall who, playing the part of Sonia, found huge fame as the star of the 1907 'Merry Widow' operetta in London. Her outfits in this show did much to promote the craze of those large hats of the Edwardian period.

known couturier – Lucy, Lady Duff Gordon (a survivor of the *Titanic* disaster), and a host of provincial establishments dotted around the country.

In 1900, it was reported that the fashion house of Lucile organised what we know today as the 'catwalk', by creating a ramp and curtained areas at one end of their London premises in Hanover Square. Here, to the accompaniment of music and lights, glamorous young ladies modelled outfits and huge feather-bedecked hats for the pleasure of invited guests. It was almost a theatrical experience in which Lucille in London (and Paul Poiret in Paris) promoted their fashions with their 'mannequin parades' which, not unsurprisingly, appealed to male audiences as working class girls had fun dressing up beyond their station in life. This sort of thing didn't suit everybody however, and in 1904, the hugely popular, but seemingly strait-laced, novelist of the time Marie Corelli complained of the 'remarkably offensive' way in which the male attendees were 'invited to stare and smile'. One can only assume that the management at Lucille were not overly happy with Marie!

Upper class hat designers and retailers such as George Bernard & Co, J M Gidding & Co, Bergdorf & Goodman and C M Phipps Inc in New York and Henry Heath and Madame Tucker Widgery in London, copiously advertised in many publications (of varying degrees of sophistication) such as the *Lady Magazine, Vogue, Women's Life,* the *London Illustrated News,* together with *Les Modes* and *La Mode Illustrée* in France, *The Illustrated Milliner* ('The American Authority on Millinery') with an annual subscription of $3 – also available in London and Paris and *The Delineator* magazine in the USA (with its magnificent fashion colour plates) to name but a few.

The American socialite and philanthropist Mollie Brown – another of the survivors of the Titanic tragedy who famously became known as 'The Unsinkable Mollie Brown' – can frequently be seen in contemporary pictures of the day sporting some of these huge creations. James Cameron's more recent epic film *Titanic* also vividly recreates a number of upper class ladies 'being seen' aboard the ship's ill fated maiden voyage wearing this type of feathered headgear shortly before at least some of them met their watery demise in 1912. Also listed in the ship's manifest as being transported, and thus lost in the sinking, was a consignment of twelve cases of ostrich plumes valued at £20,000 (equivalent to around £2 million today) and a further number of cases of 'raw feathers' also said to be on board.

And yet, disasters apart, we tend to forget that what we see as being rather quaint and old fashioned in present day terms were, in their day, considered elegant and rip-roaring up-to-date fashion – a 'must' for all the young things and well heeled socialites to have!

Goodbye 'Bertie'

Although consigned to history, I suppose there are a couple of equivalents today where one can see massive and fanciful hats on display: Ladies' Day at Ascot in the UK is one and the Kentucky Derby Festival in America is another. Similarly, George Cukor's 1964 film *My Fair Lady* offered a flavour of those marvellous creations. Even the notoriously straight laced Queen Mary and her royal entourage got in on the act, and nostalgic old photos of the swirling crowds at the earlier 1908 Franco British Exhibition staged at the White City in London (followed shortly after by the Summer Olympics of that same year) reveal that the trend for gigantic hats decorated with feathers and suchlike had really taken off – if you'll excuse the pun. The subsequent passing of Edward VII had also prompted the 'Black Ascot' race meeting in 1910 where a sea of large black hats and feathers could be seen on display as a fashionable token of respect and mourning by the great and the good for the dear departed 69-year-old scallywag. Only after Edward died did the British realise how much they had liked him. The old libertine had somehow earned the affection of his people and raised the Royal Family to new levels of popularity.

On the colonial front, old footage of the Royal visit to India – 'The Jewel in the British Crown' – by King George and Mary a year later in 1911 shows them being welcomed at a Durbar in Delhi by large crowds of local dignitaries and presumably foreign office and colonial staff with many of the ladies bedecked in these super-sized millinery creations. The local Delhi population, with barely a penny (or should I say rupee) to their names must have been somewhat taken aback to say the least at what the English 'Memsahibs' were wearing and the fashion for large hats seemed not to have spread to any great degree amongst the indigenous population – even those of higher (and thus more wealthy) castes!

The years of 'The Playboy King' Edward VII's reign were often referred to as the 'Golden Age' by some and 'La Belle Epoch' by others. After Edward's death, George V came to the throne, ushering in a more reserved era. In photographic terms, the days of the Daguerreotype, Ambrotype and the Carte de Visite were coming to an end and the humble postcard came of age – rapidly becoming the 'Twitter' of its day.

Before long, postcard collecting became a massive craze and the models pictured wearing bumper size hats were just one of the many card subjects available. By 1910, those in society who determined standards of etiquette were insisting that no 'proper'

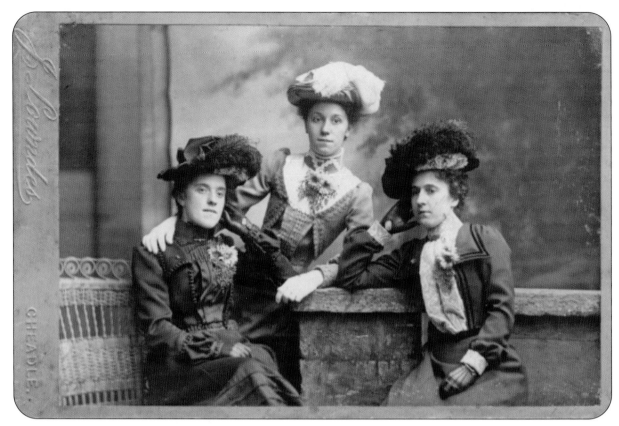

The popularity of Cartes de Visite and Cabinet cards was rapidly coming to an end. We see here, three young ladies sporting their feathered hats in this relaxed Cabinet card image from the early 1900s. *(Picture by J. Lowndes of Cheadle.)*

woman should leave the house without her head being covered by a hat! At the top end of society, Alice Keppel, one of Edward's numerous mistresses, was often seen sporting one of these giant ensembles, as could the lady members of the king's entourage at public functions and events. Depending on a woman's social standing and ability to afford them, extravagant hats were all the rage, and the fashionable ladies from the upper echelons of society who gathered around Bertie were serious contributors to this trend. Many would actually change their entire outfits several times a day – and that could involve quite a few hats! Even their parasols were often covered in expensive feathers.

Society weddings (and even those of more humble folk) during the Edwardian period also provided a great opportunity for ladies to put on the style and showcase their wonderful hat confections. Prices varied enormously and it was not unheard of for certain members of the well-heeled set (probably with more money than sense) to stump up anything towards £100 for one of these creations – an absolute fortune

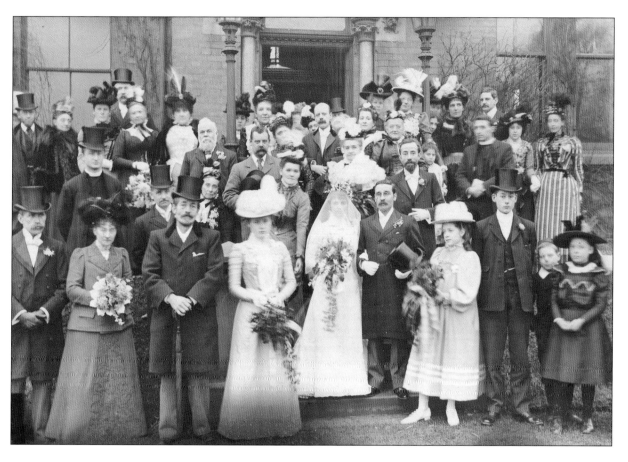

This joyful Cabinet card image, taken in Co. Antrim in 1900 depicts an array of large hats worn by the lady guests at the wedding of Alice Maud Ellen Sutton and Daniel Christie Beggs. *(Image by kind permission of Orla Fitzpatrick.)*

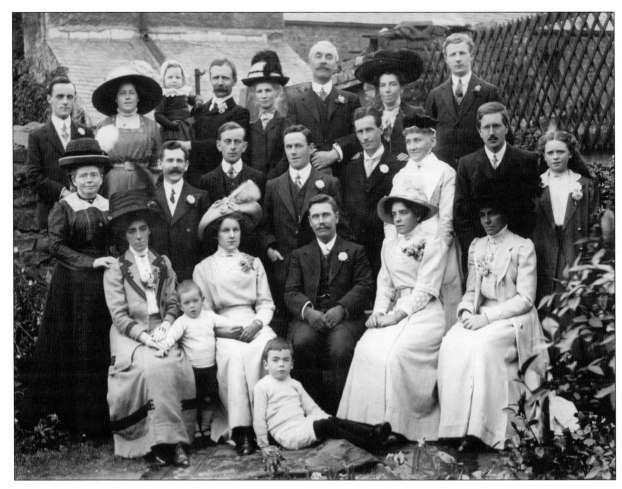

Irish Edwardian fashion to the fore with a profusion of amazing hats in this Dublin wedding picture – taken by John McCrae, circa 1910. *(Image by kind permission of Orla Fitzpatrick.)*

(over £5,000 today). Having said that, there was also a wide range of prices at the cheaper end of the market and in 1909, the Redferns establishment of London charged one customer a 'mere' five guineas for a nice little number. Likewise, also in London, The Parisian Hat Co of New Bond St., Knightsbridge and Kensington were offering 'Hats For Every Occasion – One Price Only – 30 Shillings.'

However, when you view these prices against the average annual wage of a Ladies' Maid for example, who would earn around £32 per annum, then many of these lavish hats fell way outside the scope of ordinary working class folk; even a 'mere five guineas' was, to them, an unaffordable sum. Apart from domestic service, many women were forced into low paid work such as millinery in order to supplement their husband's low wages, which often only amounted to between 12–15 shillings per week. One example from 1909 suggested that in rural Essex, some women were being paid just a pitiful 7 shillings for a long, arduous working week.

As with many new products and trends, there are spin-offs and the growth of the Edwardian fashion for bumper-sized ladies' hats meant that very large boxes were needed to store and transport them in. Many of these hatboxes were attractive in their own right, featuring beautiful graphic design work. Numerous firms got in on the act of supplying these outsized containers to the millinery trade and were doing very nicely. Women proved a very suitable, adaptable and, as mentioned in the previous paragraph, cheap source of labour in the manufacture of these boxes, which were invariably produced by hand.

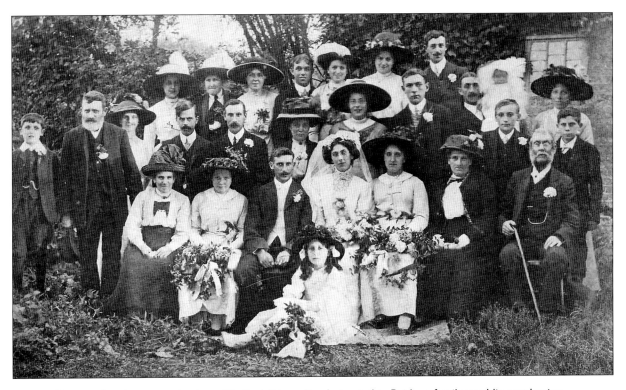

Yet another joyous gathering of ladies' Edwardian hats at this Bridges family wedding gathering. (Image by kind permission of Tommy Heywood-Briggs.)

Lucky Old Edwin

B ack in those Edwardian times, one of the main attractions of postcards was the fact that the sender didn't have to spend very much time in composing a long drawn out letter and could get away with a short précis of their 'news'. Many postcard users had various forms of personal shorthand or codings, which were only intelligible between the sender and the recipient.

Seemingly, not everybody was happy with the situation. There would, at times, be expressions of concern in the press with the *Glasgow Evening News* proffering: 'In ten years Europe will be buried beneath picture postcards.' Others suggested that the informal written styles to be found on postcards could threaten 'standards'. *The Times* proposed that some people found the use of postcards as something of an insult to the recipient and one of these, James Douglas, suggested that there were others who regarded postcards as 'vulgar and only fit for tradesmen'. On another occasion, somebody suggested that 'The picture postcard carries rudeness to the fullest extremity.'

Notwithstanding the somewhat narrow view of some, there were certain areas of concern in legal terms as governments sought to keep in check the dissemination and distribution of information across national boundaries, which was understandable during

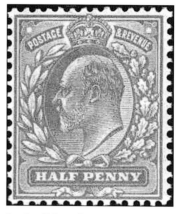

In the Edwardian era, you could send your postcard for just one halfpenny (in old money) and with up to five deliveries per day! Today's price here in 2016? A minimum of 64p and it certainly wouldn't be a same day delivery! How times change.

the years leading up to the First World War. There are also references to legal cases where postcards, or at least the information they carried, were deemed to be libellous and/or defamatory. One example of this was reported by *The Times* on 20 May 1905 when a female music teacher by the name of Melita Macready, was charged with defamatory libel, having sent the principal of the Guildhall School of Music a postcard saying – 'You old rogue, villain and liar. You old coward. Why don't you fight?' Macready was committed for trial!

Despite all the huffing and puffing from various folk, postcards, with their halfpenny stamp (as opposed to one penny for a letter), an army of postmen and five or more local deliveries per day in urban areas (with the last one sometimes being as late as 9.30 pm), were an amazingly fast method of communication and social networking in the early twentieth century; the equivalent of the 'phone call, twitter posting or text messages of today. You would not only get cards from people on holiday but, due to the speed of the service, you could actually send cards to them in return while they were still away. And for sure, it certainly helped spread fashion trends around the country astonishingly quickly. Messages on the reverse tended, in the main, to be fairly mundane offerings with birthday and Christmas wishes, the weather, 'Having a good time' at holiday locations, the state of a person's health and 'See you soon'. There was a card I found once however, from a gentleman – possibly a soldier – named Edwin. Dated 26 November 1916, it was addressed to his lady love Nellie and featured a languid, reclining nude beauty on the front (and not wearing a hat on that particular occasion!); it was very steamy indeed for the time. He openly refers to a number of things in a rather formal and florid sort of way compared to today, and among them are his lady's 'Curves of grace'. In anticipation he writes:

> *The word Remembrance seems especially nice my dearest Nellie as a descriptive one to embrace all my thoughts of those two occasions I had the delight of seeing those curves of grace. Remembrance – what a word full of meaning in all ways not only the one under discussion.*
>
> *I think for just a brief second or two on Sept 30th you looked so ravishingly nice – as the reverse portrays – though of course not to the same sweet advantage as this portrays the lady!!! You will see I had to purchase the card before learning its title – and am well pleased. It's one so appropriate for the past as well as the future.*
>
> *Remembrance of your promise of a next occasion fired with love and delight my heart towards you. As progress would suggest I will hope to see those (splendid) 'C....s' of yours still nicer than before.*
>
> *I really wish to reserve the word splendid for the spring – when I want to be able to call them splendid for their curves and for their fullness.*
>
> *If you will then allow, they shall not go away from my sight (then) without more salutations than they have heretofore received.*
>
> *From your lover – Edwin.*

As the card had no stamp and had not been franked, I assume he had rather wisely taken the decision to preserve the intimacy of the moment by sending it to Nellie inside a sealed envelope rather than giving the postman a field day and becoming the toast of the local sorting office! Edwin, obviously looking forward to even more intimate times to come and signing himself as 'Your lover' appears to have been a bit of a naughty lad!

The 'Eminence Noir'

My earliest memory of a Victorian lady in a large feathered hat was around the end of the Second World War when, as a very young lad living in my grandmother's house in war-torn Ramsgate on the Kent coast, I used to see her lodger, a very stern, and at times particularly argumentative, old lady called Miss Newby. She was a complete throwback to that earlier generation, as she determinedly made the ascent to her rented apartment way up on the top floor, climbing the steep, creaky stairs in her high black lace-up boots, long black dress, black shawl and, of course, a large black hat with black and white feathers! Looking back she seemed, to my childlike imagination, to be like one of Charles Dickens' darker characters or, at the very least, dressed for a funeral. I kept my distance from this sinister presence, this spooky 'Eminence Noir' and with Miss Newby around, who needed the Luftwaffe!

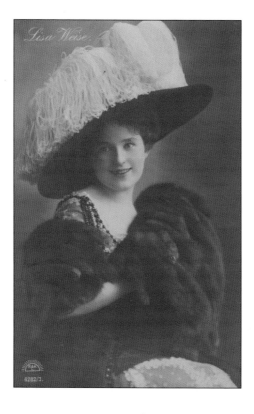

Sleepers

That said, and despite past memories of Miss Newby, little did I realise that, thirty-five years or so later, and purely by chance, I would develop a firm interest in images of Edwardian ladies wearing large feathered hats!

Back in the mid-1970s, I really had no interest in the subject at all but it was a chance visit to the local postcard club in Norwich that changed all that. It was one of their monthly meetings and while browsing through some of the 1000s of cards

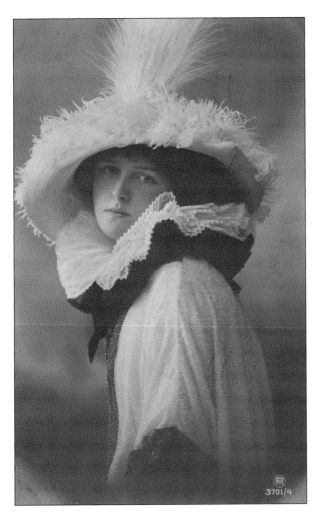

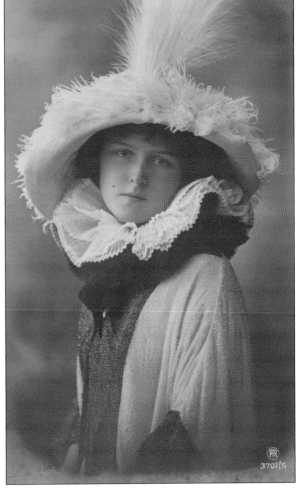

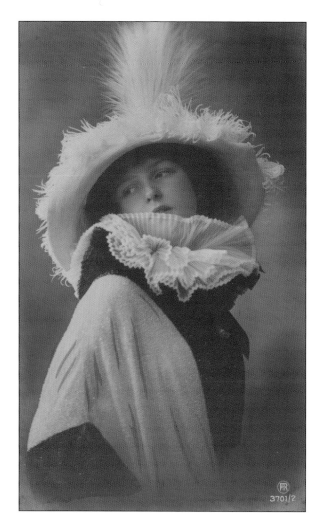

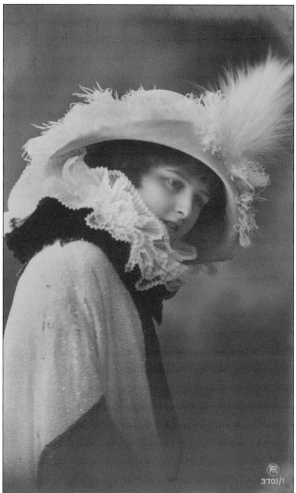

on offer, I was approached by the club chairman who welcomed me and asked about my collecting interests. I had to admit to having none but asked what he, the expert, would recommend. He took me to one side and produced a beautiful complete set of six cards featuring a very attractive young lady in various poses wearing a large feathered hat.

'What do you think of these?' he asked, 'These are what we call "sleepers" and nobody really wants them at present. You can have this whole set for 90p'.

Ninety pence? A mere ninety pence for the whole set? It seemed far too good a deal to miss. My collection was under way and even all these years later, this first beautifully tinted set is still one of my favourites.

Following my purchase, the postcard-collecting bug had bitten and my journey had begun. I was hooked on these period lovelies and have been ever since, with cards sourced from the UK, Belgium, Austria, Holland, France, across Europe in general and of course the good old USA where, not surprisingly, postcards featuring large 'showy' hats are also very popular.

Amusingly, subsequent visits to the Norwich postcard club led me to dealings with a real local character by the name of Ronnie Rouse. The rotund Ronnie was a small-time postcard, cigarette card and ephemera dealer who, for whatever reason, usually dressed himself in a Sherlock Holmes type 'deerstalker' hat complemented by a tent-like heavy old overcoat that almost reached the ground. Quite a sight! However, there was a certain underlying problem. Our intrepid dealer had an aversion to soap and water and although he invariably seemed to have a nice selection of 'hats' cards on offer, all dealings with him as far as I was concerned, had to be done at arm's length – and quickly! I well remember the time when Ronnie was stuck for a lift home at the end of the evening and asked me if I could oblige. My heart sank.

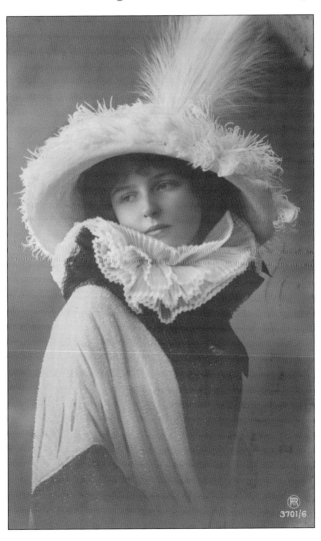

There followed an extremely odorous three-mile journey back to his place – a terraced house at the top of a steep hill crammed with postcards and numerous other antique 'goodies'. You could hardly push the door open such was his acquisitive nature! The favour completed, the trip back to my own place was undertaken with all the windows in the car firmly open. A lingering memory never to be forgotten!

Whilst today, some rare category postcards can fetch very large sums, prices for the 'sleepers' in my early 'Hat' collecting days often ranged from 10p to 20p each – ridiculously low when you think that today, some of those self same 'Glamour' cards, depending on scarcity, condition and aesthetic value, can sometimes run into several pounds each. The 'sleepers' it appears are 'sleepers' no longer.

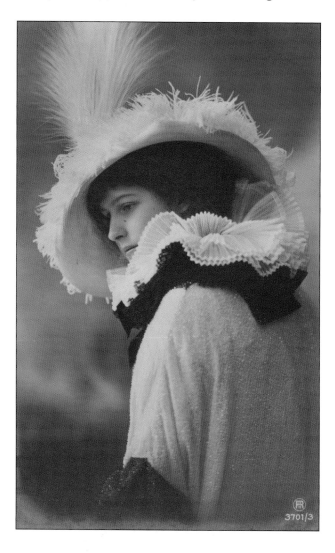

Rose Tinted Spectacles

B ut why my interest in these ladies and their hats you might ask? Well, as a traditionalist and historian, all I can think of as an excuse is that they are so evocative of that long-gone period of our history leading up to the Great War. A period which, thanks to the benefit of rose tinted spectacles, seems a gentler and much more elegant age – at least for those with money and status within a rigid and entrenched class structure. For some reason, the Edwardian era, (possibly due to the many period dramas on TV, particularly the popular *Downton Abbey*), has managed to leave us with visual impression of a sort of romantic golden age; warm sunny afternoons; the hunting, shooting and fishing set in their tweeds; genteel social events such as Royal Ascot and Henley Regatta; the mellow glow of Empire and naughty

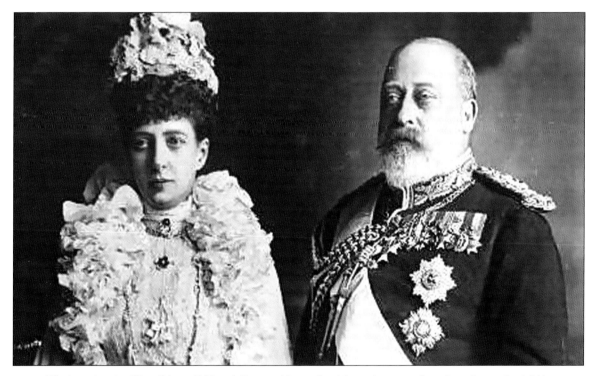

Their majesties King Edward VII and Queen Alexandra. Note the queen's rather distant look. Was she perhaps contemplating her husband's numerous affairs or perhaps remembering Denmark?

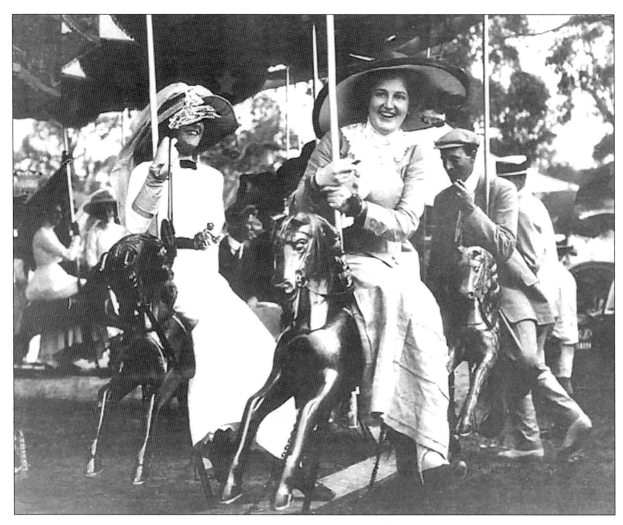

On the far side of the world, large hats, not surprisingly, had also become all the rage. Pictured here at the Deepwater Races in New South Wales, Australia in 1910, we see two smiling ladies (giant hats firmly in place!) as they take a spin on a local fun fair ride.

Bertie having fun with his ladies. For the poor and lower classes however, it was a very different scenario.

Whatever the true realities of Edward VII's reign, it seems almost absurd to us in the early twenty-first century that these beautiful young ladies walked around in those often huge Edwardian UFO sized hats – smothered with feathers and various other animal trimmings – (once referred to as 'zoological decoration'), without batting an eyelid. And yet all those grainy old films and newsreels of the day show us that's exactly what they did – and went about their business without a second thought.

However, there were certain everyday problems. As an example, the traditional music halls flourished during the Edwardian period and, as a patron, you would certainly not want to find yourself seated behind one of these 'dedicated followers of fashion' in her large and obtrusive hat. Having said that, and to be fair to the theatres themselves, many insisted that lady patrons remove them – which for some was no mean feat. Similarly, any attempt at a furtive kiss from some ardent young admirer must have proved problematic! Have a look at any old movie film of the period, such as those to be found in the Huntley Film Archives or British Pathe for instance, and it can be very difficult to pick out a lady in any upmarket Edwardian street full of people who is not wearing a hat of some shape or size. What those wearing ultra large ones did on really windy days, or being driven around in the newly fashionable motor cars, or sitting in an open-topped tram, heaven only knows, but such is fashion and in good old British tradition, they coped!

One account by a certain Minna Irvine related the problems with motoring in 1909 when she recounted: '…before I had been riding half an hour. I discovered that motoring discourages all the vanities of fashion. As soon as the machine gathered speed, the wind whipped my coat open and tore off my hat!'

Notwithstanding the odd passing difficulty, and to combat the 'motoring' problem to some degree, veils were introduced to secure the hat in place, protect the hair and keep out at least some of the dust while on the road. Some enterprising retailers, seizing the moment, also went as far as advertising their hats as 'Suitable for Motoring'. An image from 1909 also shows one couple, with the lady wearing her 'motoring' style hats, taking their marriage vows and tying the knot in a balloon high over New York! Ballooning and balloon racing had become very popular in Edwardian era and another image, also from 1909, shows the large field at the swanky Hurlingham Club in London, full of large gas-filled balloons and, even fuller still, with large numbers of fashionable (and presumably pretty well off) lady spectators in their large feather covered headwear waiting for the spectacle of the take offs.

The following pages, feature images of an amazing range of ladies feathered hats, a number of which were possibly included in various copies of The Queen magazine during the Edwardian period. They give the reader a first-hand taste of how this particular fashion craze had captured the imagination of both the upper and lower classes within society and the female public in general. Similar images were to be found in various notable fashion magazines of the period such as La Mode Illustrée in France.

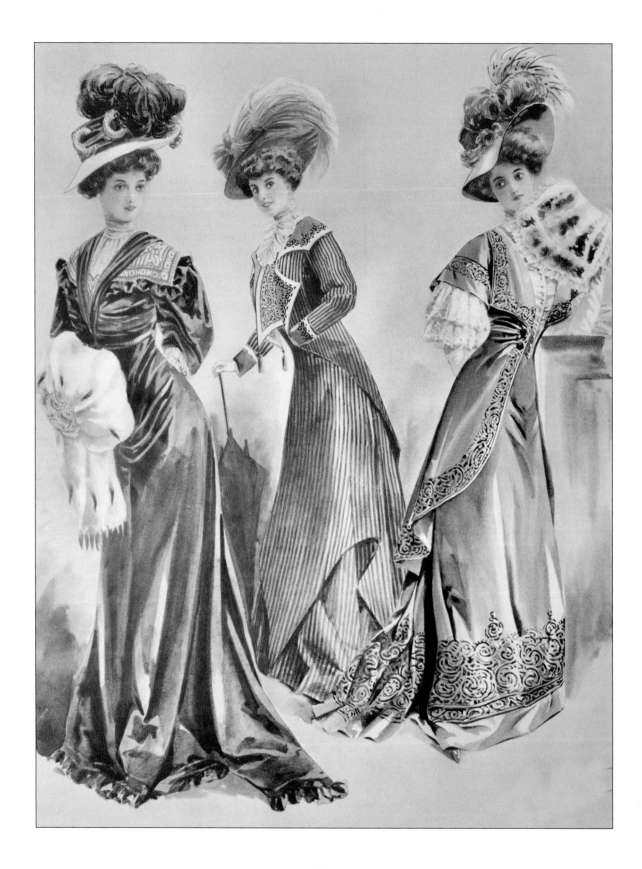

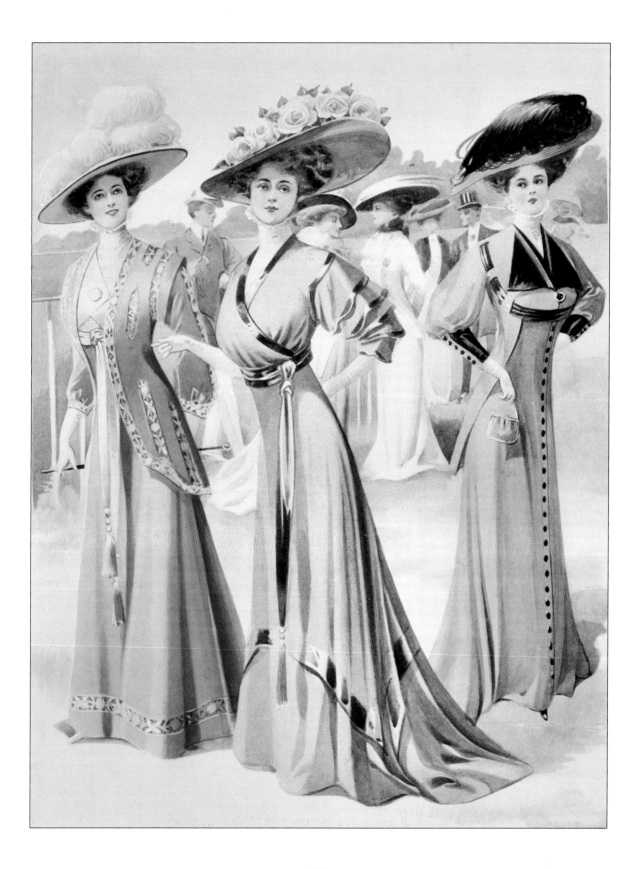

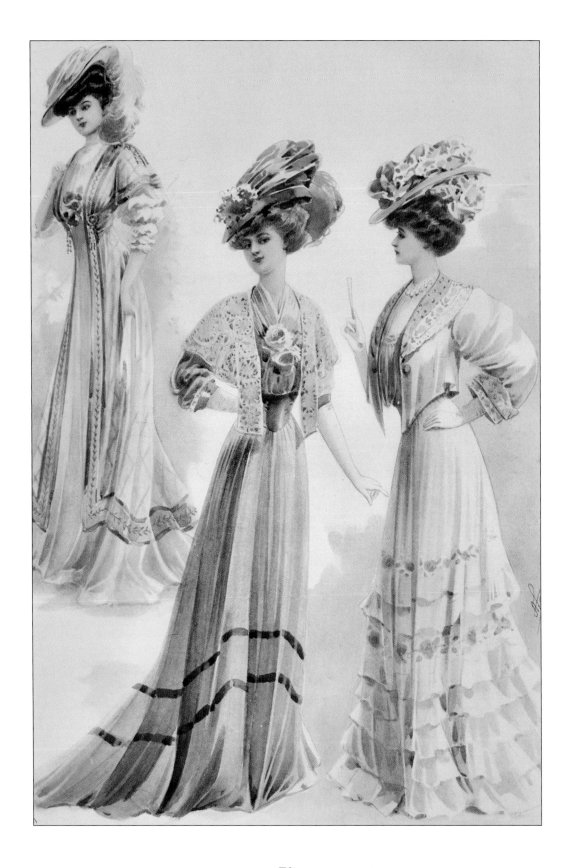

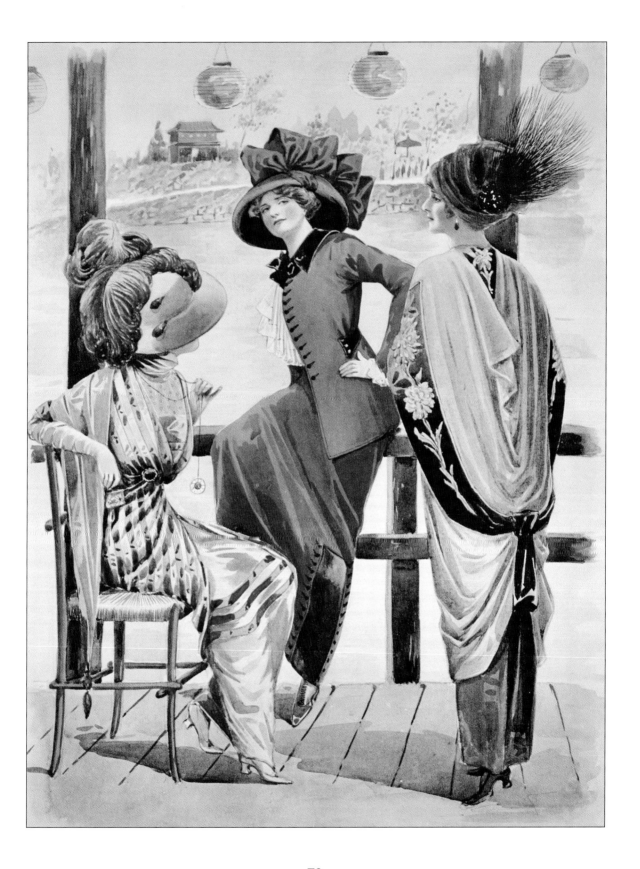

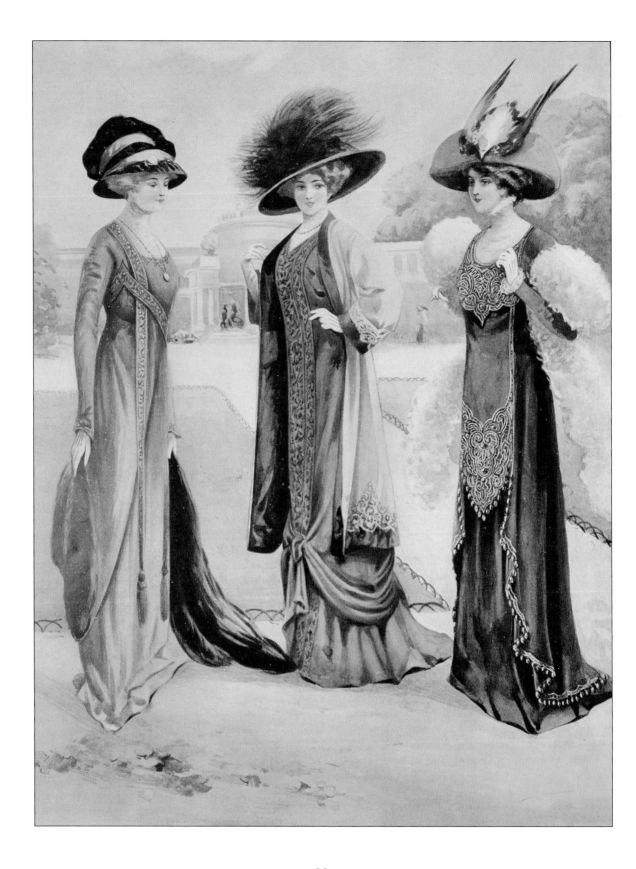

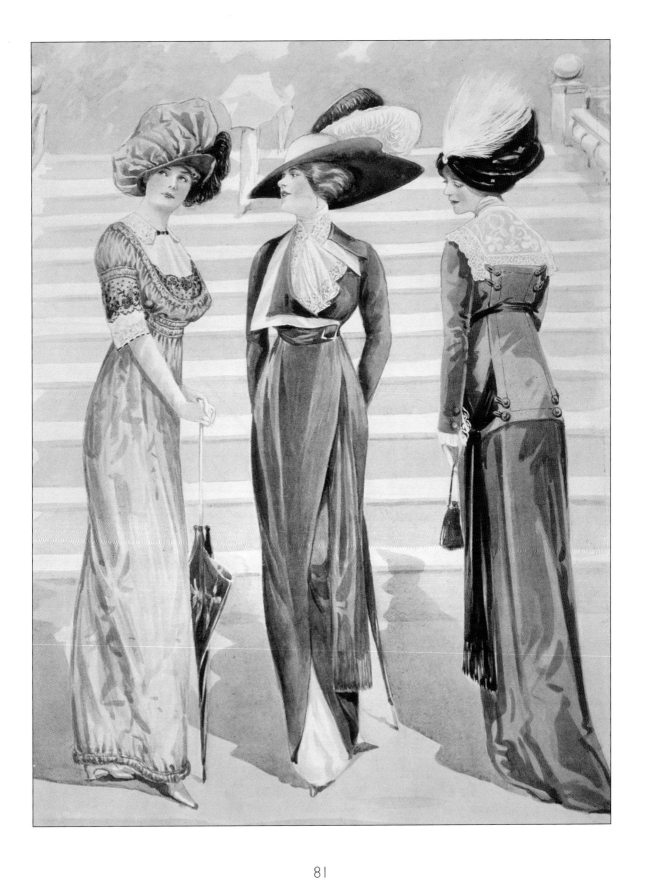

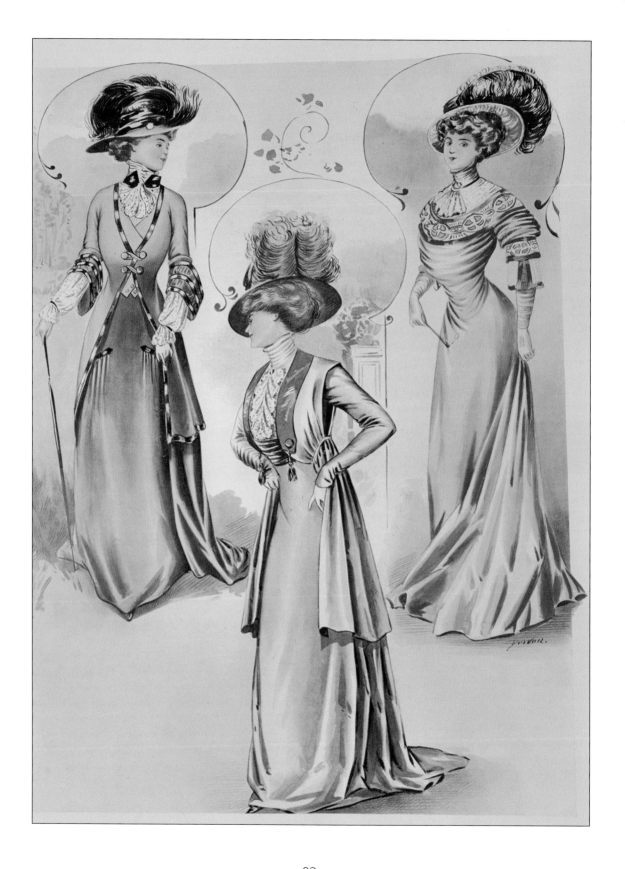

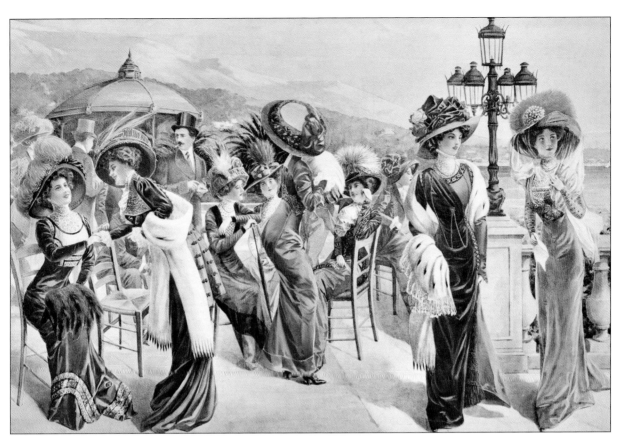

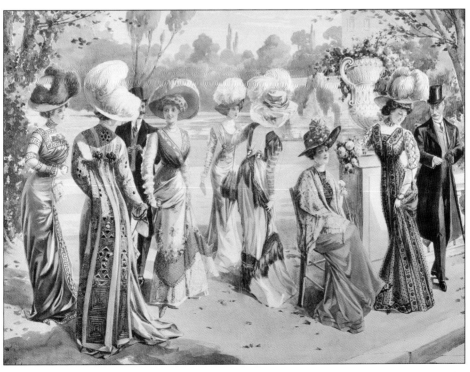

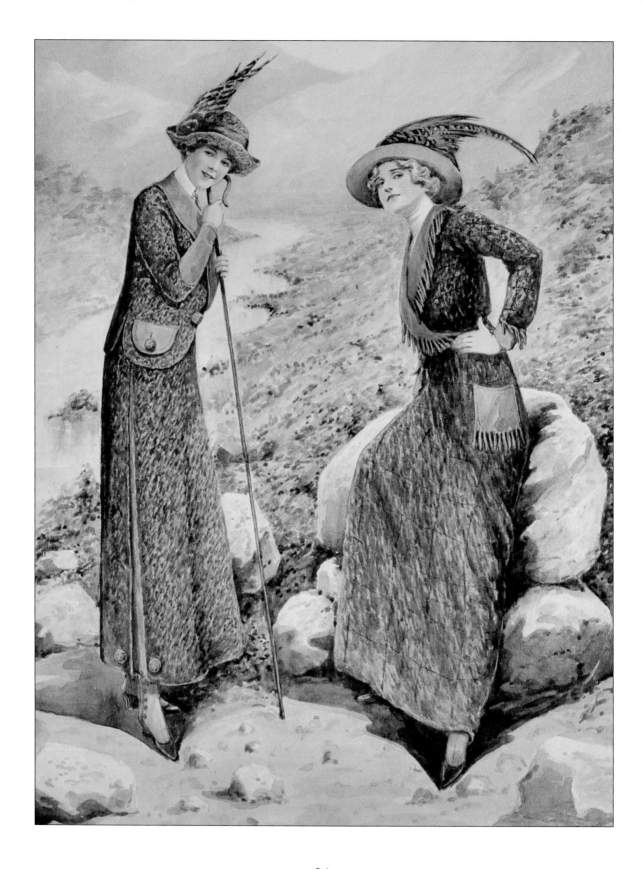

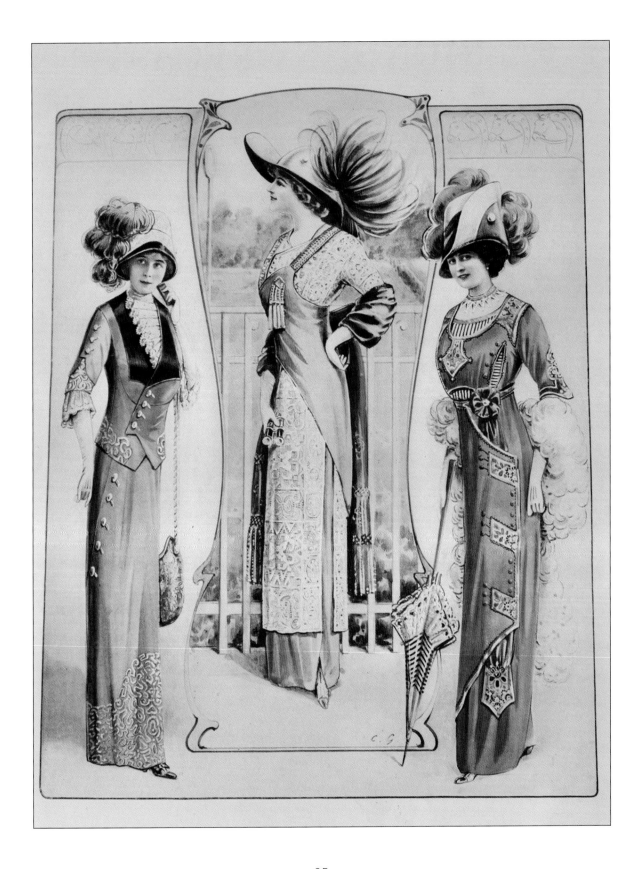

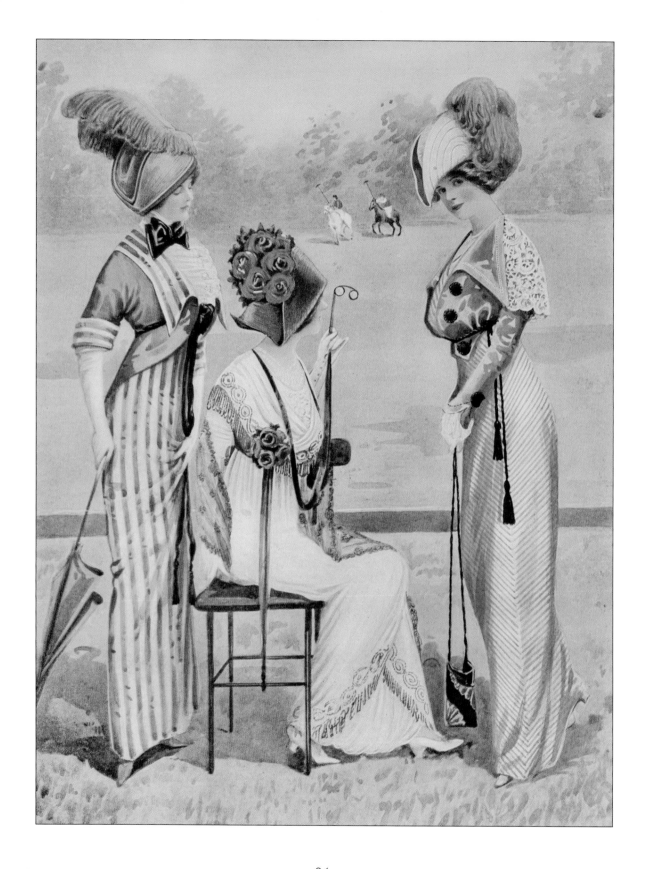

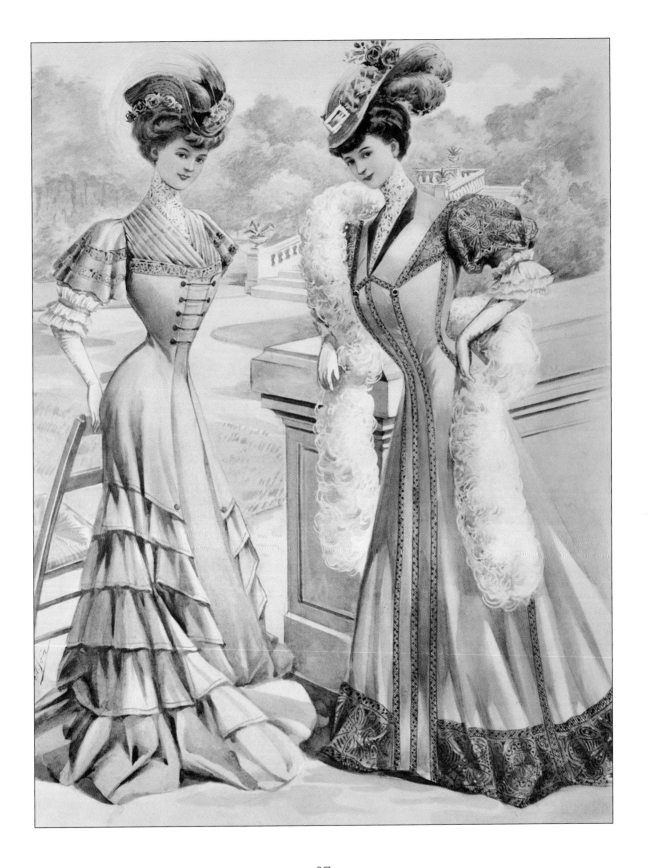

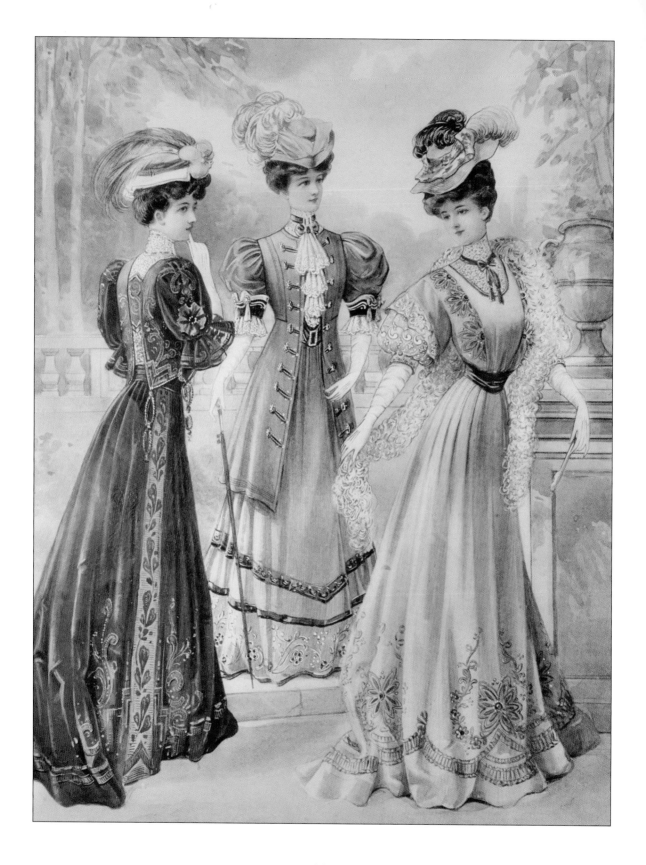

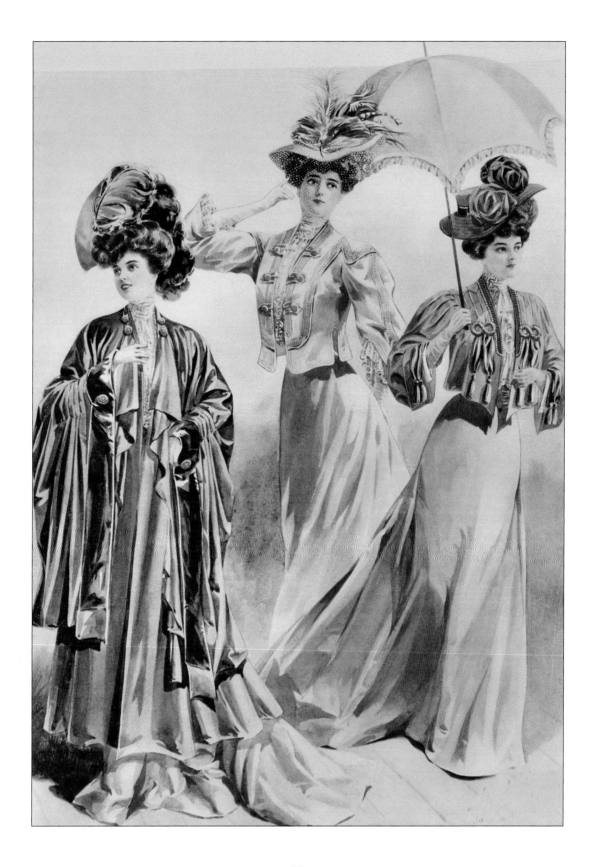

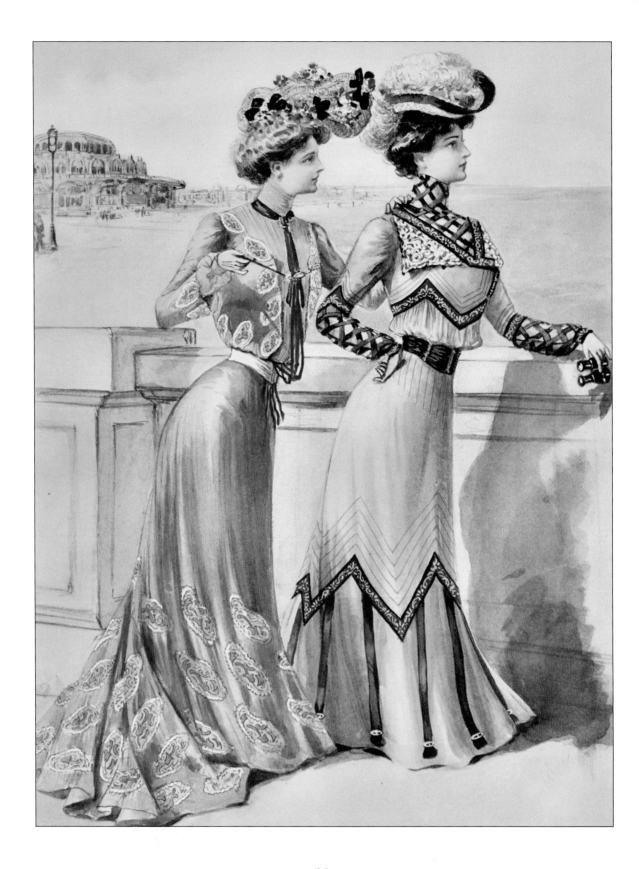

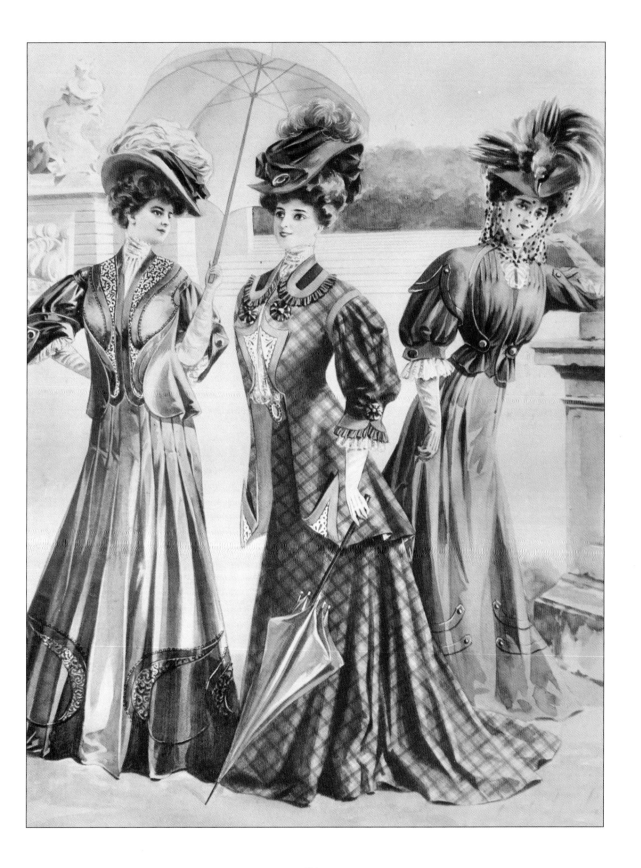

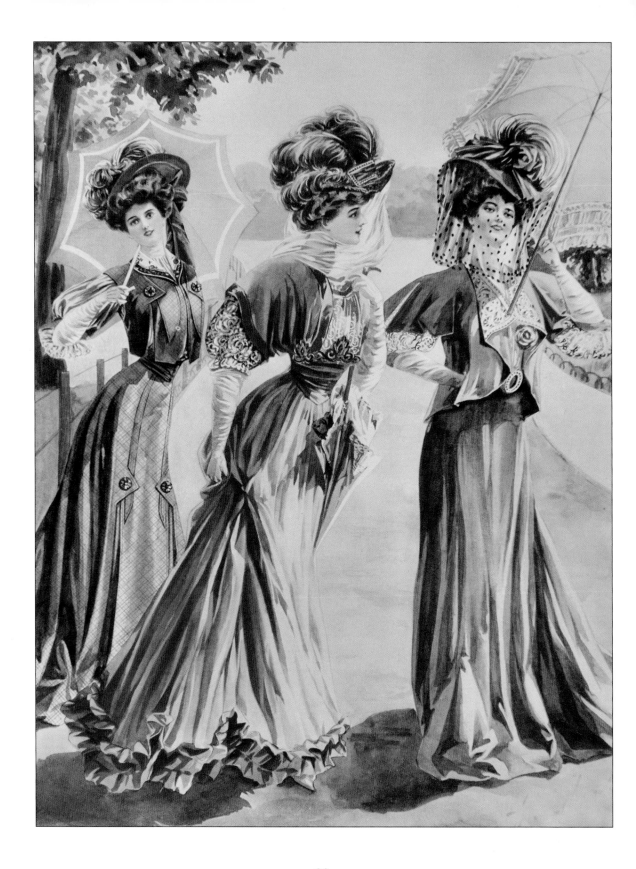

Escape to the Seaside

The development of the railways during the Victorian and Edwardian eras meant that for city dwellers, and at reasonable cost, getting to the coast had become a much easier proposition for those seeking 'freedom'. Superb railway posters, much sought after today, appeared all over the place exhorting people to hop on the train. This was a chance to get away from it all and escape from the claustrophobia of the city. The seaside had become the place to go.

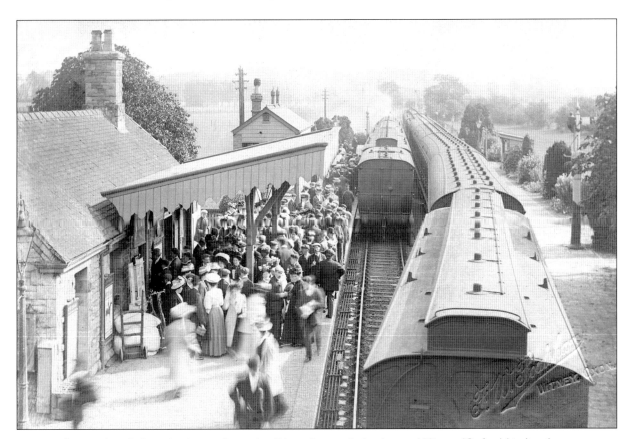

A typical and charming image from the Edwardian period, taken at Witney (Oxfordshire) railway station in around 1908. Note the profusion of ladies in large hats as the crowd jostles to purchase their tickets for an away day to the coast. Due to the slow exposure of the photograph, one can also see some 'ghost' like figures scurrying around on the platform. *(Image by courtesy of Martin Loader.)*

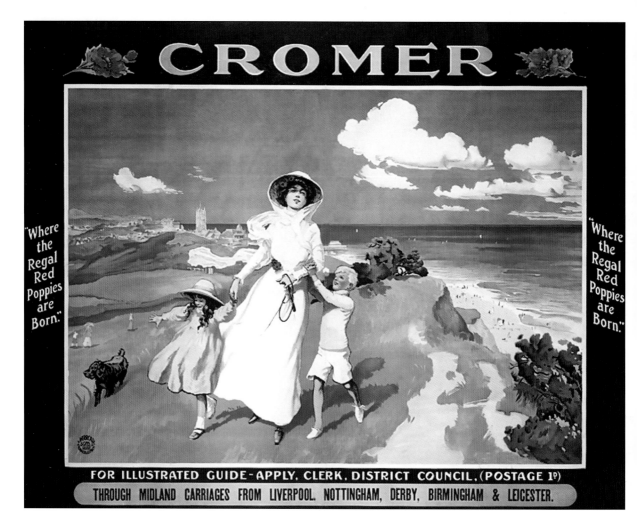

CROMER

"Where the Regal Red Poppies are Born."

"Where the Regal Red Poppies are Born."

FOR ILLUSTRATED GUIDE - APPLY, CLERK, DISTRICT COUNCIL, (POSTAGE 1ᵈ)

THROUGH MIDLAND CARRIAGES FROM LIVERPOOL, NOTTINGHAM, DERBY, BIRMINGHAM & LEICESTER.

Large hats even got in on the act as depicted on this charming Cromer railway tourist poster with a mother and her two children strolling along the windy North Norfolk cliff tops.

As a result, numerous seaside resorts benefitted from a massive influx of visitors. Landladies and boarding-house keepers at popular places such as Blackpool, Brighton, Whitby in Yorkshire and Great Yarmouth would have had a field day. In Scotland, Ayr too became something of a magnet, especially for many Glaswegians escaping their sombre tenements. Trips to the 'Med' and flights to sunny climes, which we nowadays take for granted were, of course, unheard of for these eager visitors.

Search through any pile of early twentieth century postcards and there is more than an even chance that you will turn up numerous examples of seaside images featuring vast swathes of Edwardian folk strutting their stuff along the promenades, with the men, more often than not, sporting 'natty' boaters and the ladies tucked in under their massive hats.

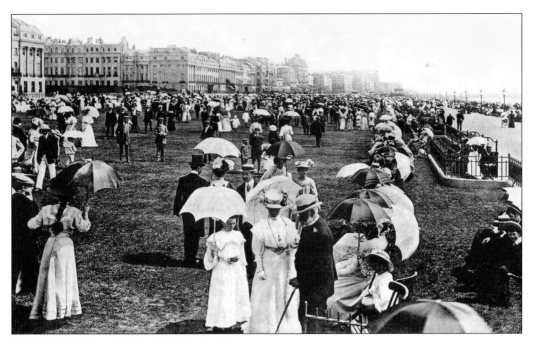

The Brunswick Lawns area of Hove, on England's south coast, illustrates just how large ladies hats had caught on as the crowds strutted their stuff along the promenade.

Late Edwardian times and this wonderful image shows a wealth of street detail and visitors crowding aboard a Blackpool tram to take the 'Circular Tour' around the resort. Note how almost every person (especially the ladies) in the picture is wearing a hat. *(Image by courtesy of Brian Turner.)*

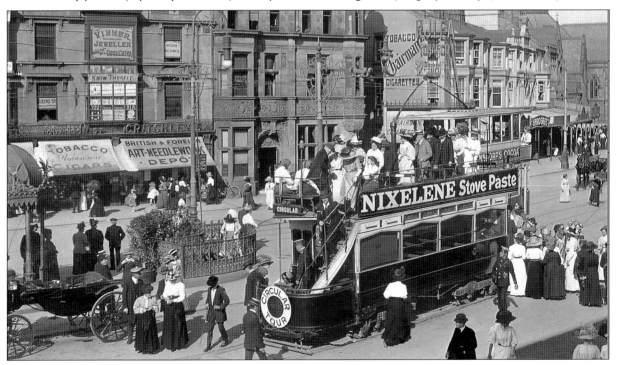

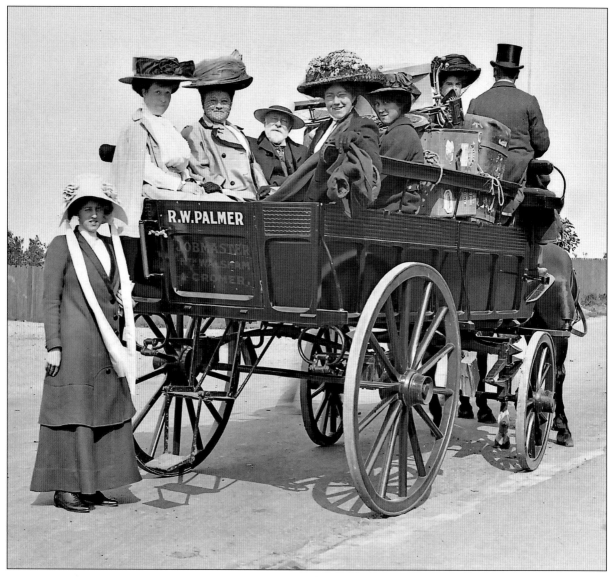

On the North Norfolk coast, the Sheringham of the Edwardian period was a very trendy and socially upmarket place. In this delightful image, taken by Cecil Hewitt in the summer of 1910, we see members of his well-to-do family, with the ladies dressed to the nines in their large, extravagant hats – being transported to Sheringham railway station by a horse drawn carriage. *(Image by kind permission of the Mo Museum, Sheringham, Norfolk.)*

Opposite: Even splashing about in the shallows, the ubiquitous large hat was never far away although this particular image, obviously retouched, probably from an Edwardian postcard, is a studio mock-up. Seagulls in the studio could have proved just a touch difficult!

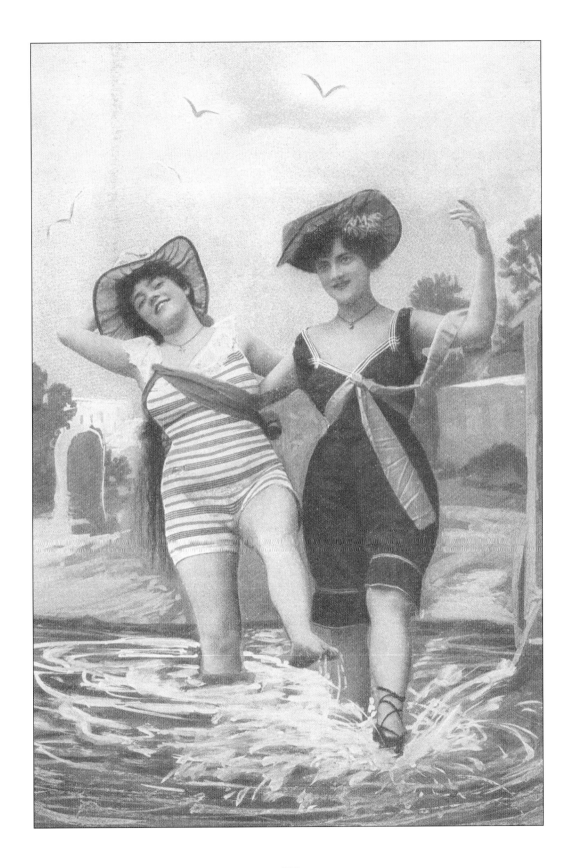

Today, visit any of the more popular modern seaside resorts and one will see the usual assortment of colourful shorts, bikinis, sunglasses and casual wear etc, but a hundred years ago in those more formal times, it was a very different story. The aforementioned postcards often show great masses of people strolling along the promenades and piers, perhaps taking a carriage ride and maybe making a trip around the bay on a paddle steamer. For the ladies, this was a chance to show off those super-sized hats in what were amazing seaside fashion displays. They were everywhere.

On crowded beaches, ladies could be seen strolling on the sands in full-length dresses, topped off with the ubiquitous, large and expansive hats. Sunglasses for the ladies were not altogether established but, had they been commonplace in those days, they would have been superfluous because the hats themselves provided more than enough shade with their enormous brims! And when parading the seafront became a little arduous, one could resort to deckchairs, Punch and Judy, various amusements and perhaps a 'Penny–Lick'* ice cream. Today, this laid back scenario seems like a different world which in reality of course, it was.

---

* 'Penny-Licks' were small, thick, clear glasses of ice cream, which folks could purchase for one penny from the sellers along the sea front. The customer would lick the ice cream from the glass, returning the empty to the seller. With the minimum of cleansing, the glass would immediately be refilled for the next customer. It didn't take too many years for this practice to be banned on grounds of hygiene, resulting in the edible cones we know today.

Edward Linley Sambourne

But while all these ladies were strutting their stuff in their pretty and voluminous hats around town, city and seaside, little did some of them realise that they were being surreptitiously watched – but by whom? Fortunately, no one with sinister intentions!

Edward Linley Sambourne (1844 – 1910), an artist and illustrator, who was later to become chief cartoonist for the *Punch* magazine was frequently to be seen 'prowling' the streets of Edwardian London and, later, Paris – in the nicest possible way of course. Like many artists and illustrators even today, Sambourne in the late 1800s and early 1900s resorted to photographic reference for his figure work as a cartoonist. The difference between Sambourne and just about all the other photographers of the day was that he shot many of his pictures in secret in a sort of late Victorian and Edwardian Candid Camera scenario with what must have been a pretty small camera for the times. Difficult to secrete away a big plate camera you might imagine, and no digital stuff for our Edward, but having said that, there were some fairly small innovatively disguised cameras around at that time. It is in his 'secret' pictures, several of which are featured in this book, that we see the ladies of the day in a completely informal way, un-posed, and relaxed in their large hats going about

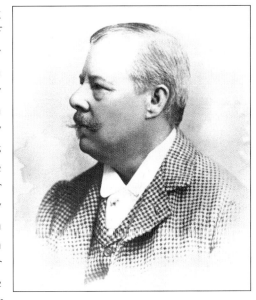

The talented Edward Linley Sambourne 1844-1910 – illustrator, amateur photographer and one time chief-cartoonist for *Punch* magazine in London. (*Image by kind permission of The Royal Borough of Kensington & Chelsea.*)

their daily lives. One can imagine that there must have been a few awkward occasions when his cover was blown in those rather more formal times and that must have been a bit tricky. But nonetheless, his interesting images confirm once again the hold that these amazing hats had on the ladies of the day.

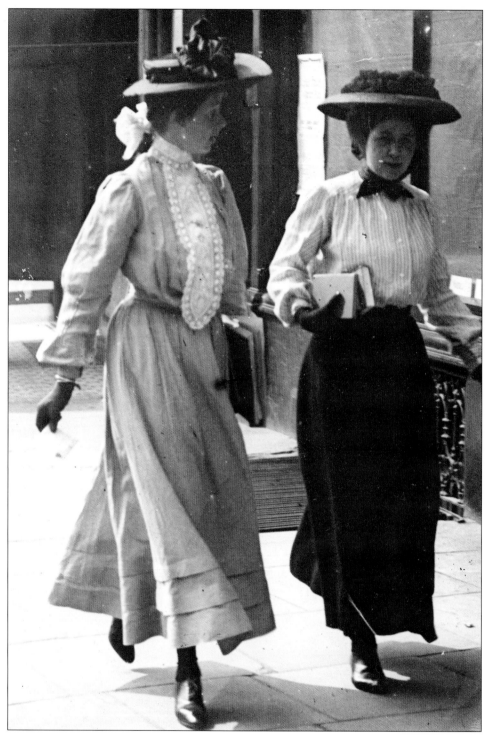

Edward Linley Sambourne: In this shot, Sambourne captures two ladies carrying books and in deep discussion as they stroll through Kensington, London on 4 July 1906. (*Image by kind permission of The Royal Borough of Kensington & Chelsea.*)

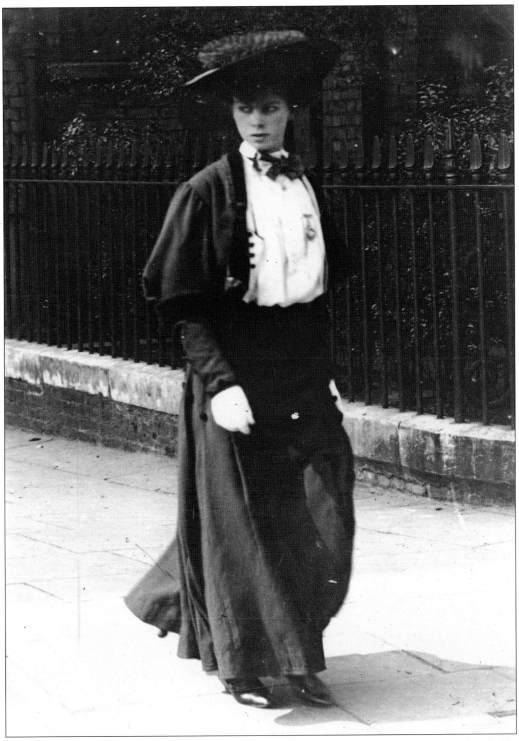

Edward Linley Sambourne: An enquiring, seemingly cautious, sideways look is given by this darkly dressed young lady as she strolls along the Cromwell Road, London on 19 June 1906. (*Image by kind permission of The Royal Borough of Kensington & Chelsea.*)

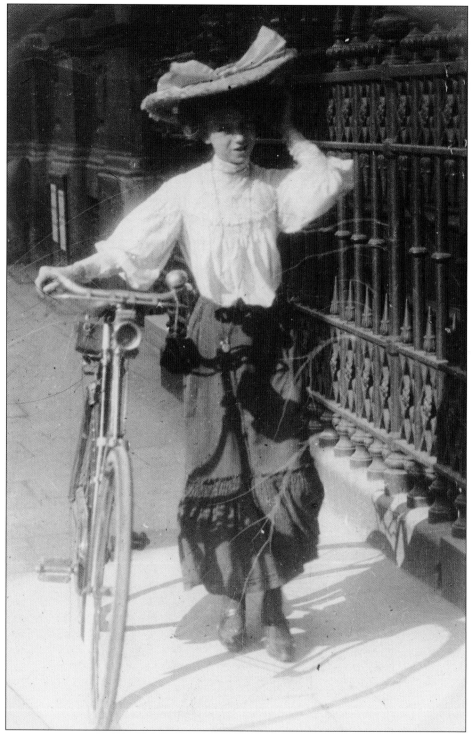

Edward Linley Sambourne: A female cyclist adjusts her large hat. Quite a feat to ride a bike wearing one of those! Picture taken in Kensington on 8 September 1906. (*Image by kind permission of The Royal Borough of Kensington & Chelsea.*)

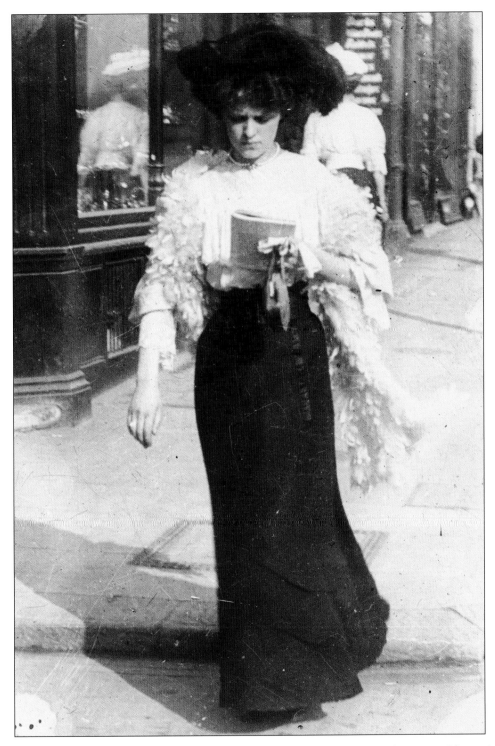

Edward Linley Sambourne: Another young lady who Sambourne describes as a 'shop girl', engrossed in her book as she strolls along Church Street, Kensington, London on 8 September 1906. (*Image by kind permission of The Royal Borough of Kensington & Chelsea.*)

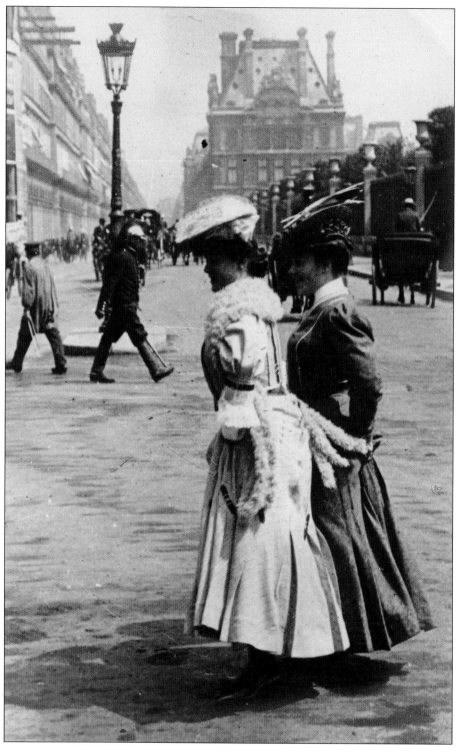

Edward Linley Sambourne: A pair of pretty young ladies enjoying the atmosphere somewhere in Paris on 3 June 1906. (*Image by kind permission of The Royal Borough of Kensington & Chelsea.*)

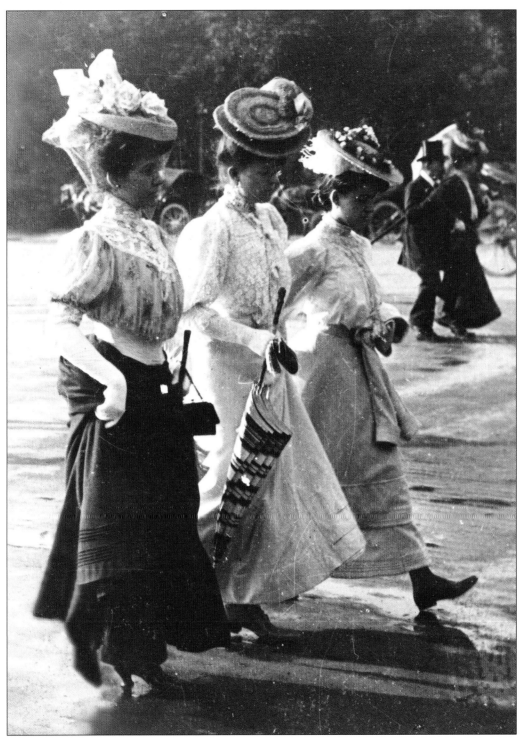

Edward Linley Sambourne: What a glamorous and chic trio. Picture taken by Sambourne in the Champs Elysees, Paris – 3 June 1906. (*Image by kind permission of The Royal Borough of Kensington & Chelsea.*)

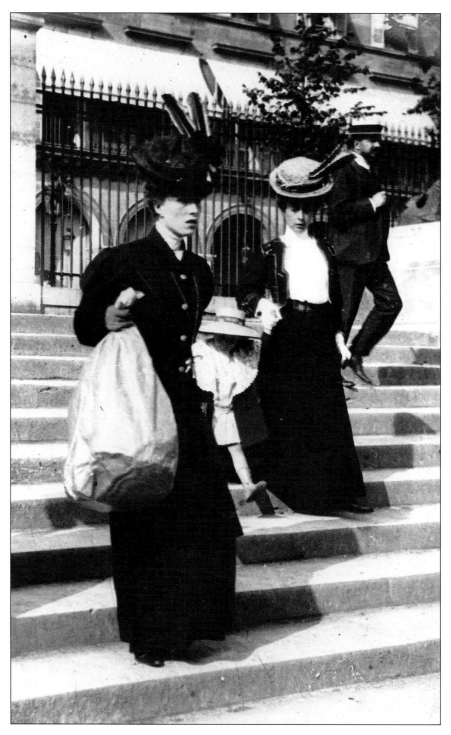

Edward Linley Sambourne: 'Mind that Step!' Taken in the Rue de Rivoli, Paris, on 5 June 1906. This package-laden lady with her companion and child make their way down the steps. Not the easiest of tasks in those voluminous skirts, but interesting hats! (*Image by kind permission of The Royal Borough of Kensington & Chelsea.*)

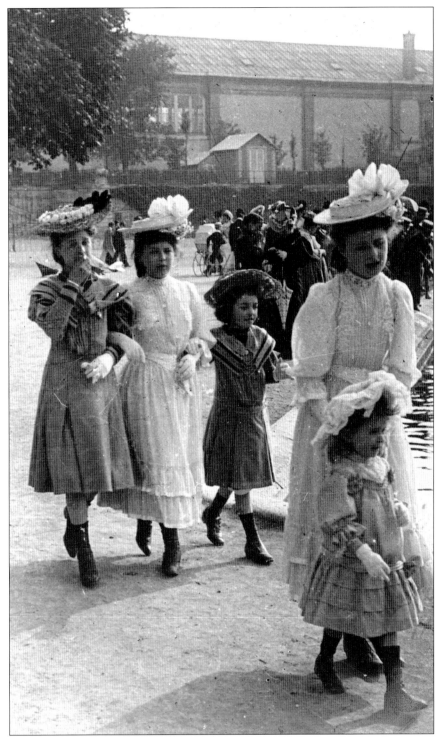

Edward Linley Sambourne: The Tuileries Gardens, Paris – 4 June 1906. Looks like a family day out around the pond. Even the young children have delightful little hats. (*Image by kind permission of The Royal Borough of Kensington & Chelsea.*)

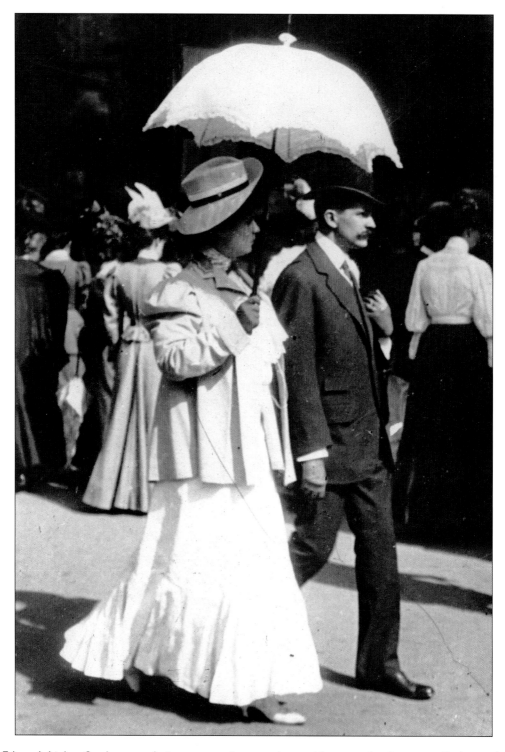

Edward Linley Sambourne: A jaunty couple, complete with parasol take a stroll down the Boulevard des Italiens, Paris – 5 June 1906. (*Image by kind permission of The Royal Borough of Kensington & Chelsea.*)

Hatpins

Many Edwardian hat creations were seemingly more of an event than an item of headgear and a spin off from these enormous hats was that from around 1902, aided by supports called 'Pompadour' frames (constructed from natural wavy hair and something of a hangover from Victorian times), around which the ladies' hair was gathered and worked in, and often supplemented with pads called 'rats' to bolster the hair. On top of this, whole ranges of beautiful hatpins were developed with many featuring ornate decorations at the non-pointed end. The creative people within the hatpin industry really went to town producing beautiful little works of art. Birmingham became the main UK production centre for these accessories along with firms like Charles Horner of Halifax.

Today, there is an enduring interest in Edwardian hatpins around the world and the following images of amazing examples are reproduced by kind permission of Leslie Woodbury of the American Hat Pin Society and Paul Moorehead of the Hat Pin Society of Great Britain respectively.

There follows an amazing array of beautiful hatpin decorations from both America and the UK. One can only admire the skill, flare and creativity which came into play in the production of these stunning fashion accoutrements.

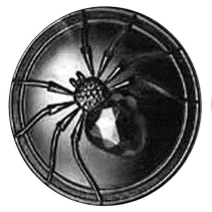
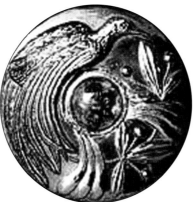
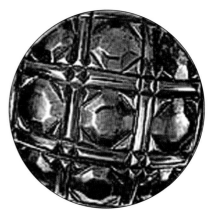

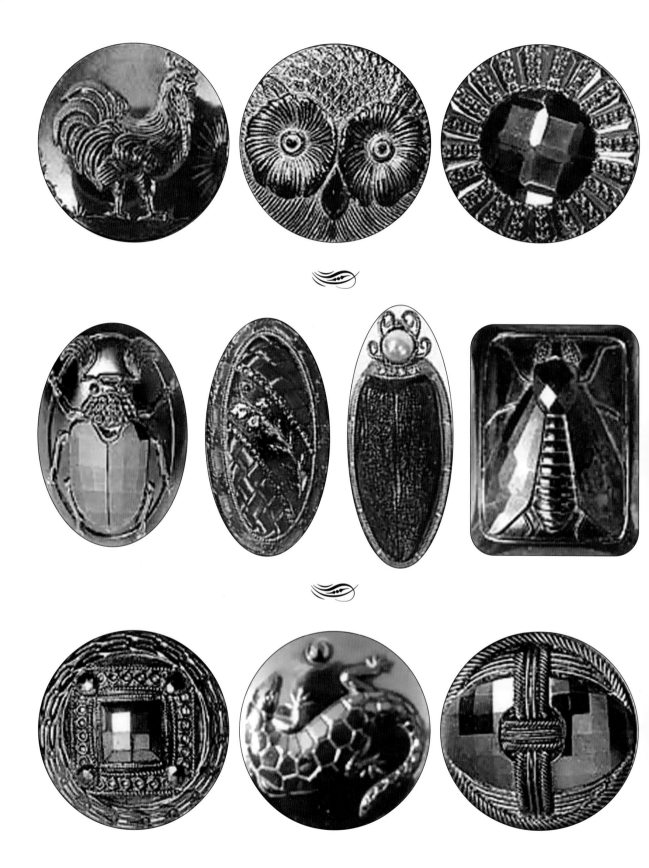

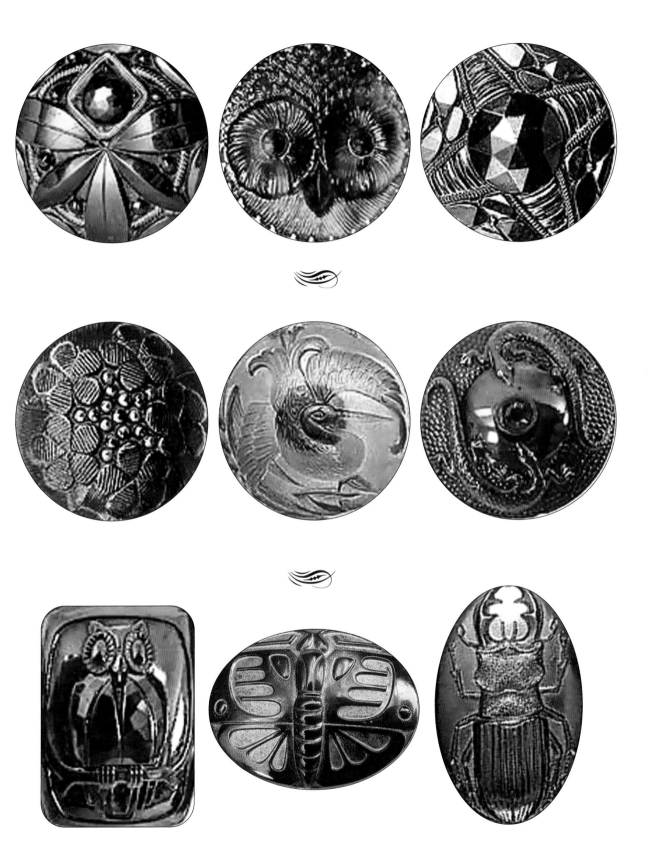

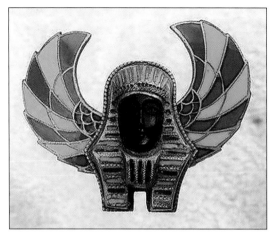

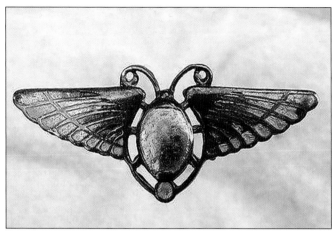

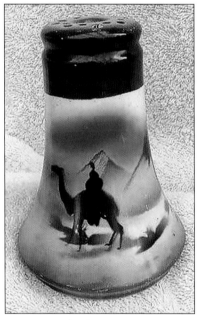

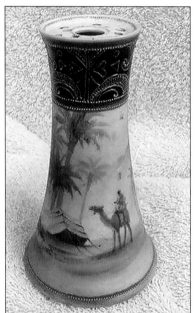

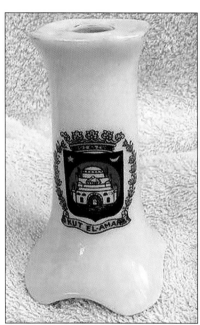

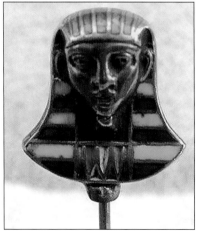

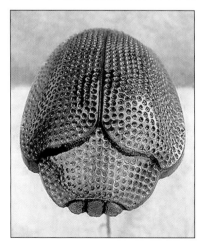

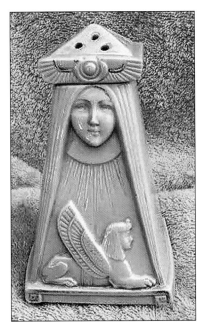

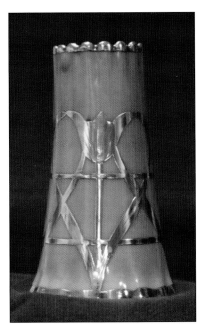

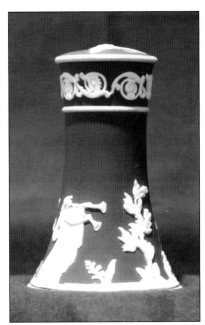

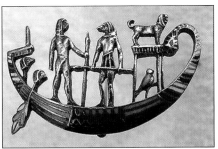

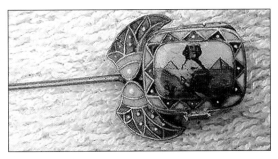

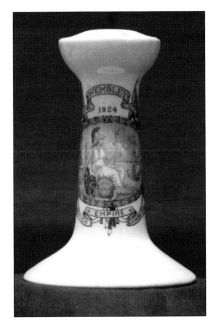

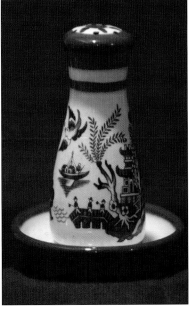

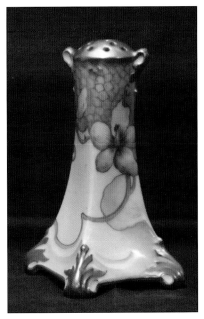

Wilhelm Staerz of Czechoslovakia and the long established Abel Morrall Ltd of Redditch – were long time manufacturers of various sorts of needles. Japan too, never a country to miss the half chance, whilst not wearing hatpins themselves, saw an opportunity and made a commercial contribution to what was on offer – becoming an established supplier of the ceramic decorated hatpin embellishments which, at the time, were known as 'Satsuma' style and often featured figures of geishas and suchlike. America too, with a population of over eighty million in 1905, was carried away by the hat boom and with a hat crazy population of that size, there was business to be done. Quite a few US manufacturers sprung up such as Unger Bros. Amgel, Lincoln, Alvin Manufacturing, The Sterling Company, William Kerr, Day & Clarke, and R. Blackington & Co together with quite a few smaller manufacturers in the Massachusetts region.

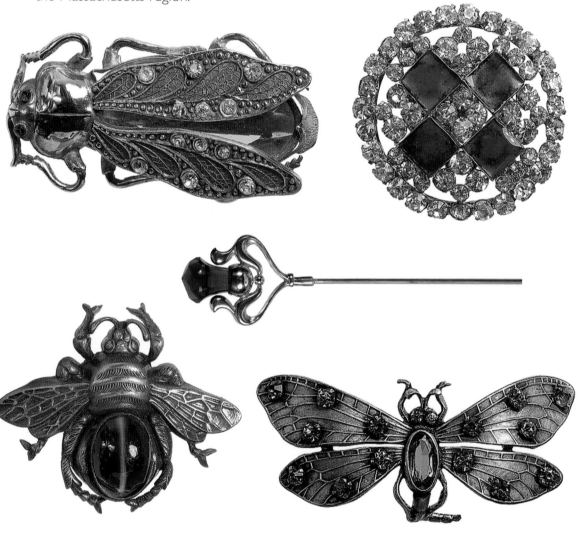

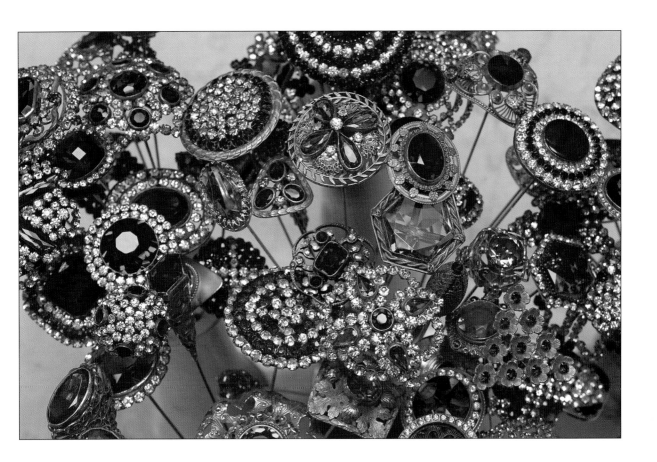

Around the world, one could find the work of superb hatpin designers coming to the fore with the likes of Barton Jenks, James Wooley, William Codman, George Gebelein and probably the greatest of them all – Louis Tiffany.

On the near continent, the Paris companies of Lalique and Fabergé were both involved with the manufacture/supply of the finest quality, top of the range hatpins. That said, there were also many pins imported from Bohemia in general with the hatpin heads featuring a multitude of materials such as gold, silver, cloisonné, mother of pearl, Viennese enamel and even insects. Some even had tiny peep-scope devices (very much along the lines of the old Victorian 'Stanhopes') offering scenic views such as Niagara Falls while others, more politically motivated, featured images of suffragettes. The choice was enormous. On the subject of suffragettes, who can forget the old British Pathe film scenes at the Epsom Derby on 4 June 1914 when Emily Davidson was mortally injured while attempting to make a political protest as she ran in front of George V's racehorse Anmer; to see her large hat rolling forlornly across the grass moments after the collision is poignant indeed.

The Sting of a Hornet

Many of these hatpins were so attractive (and often extremely expensive) that they have become a specific field of collecting in their own right. The fact that they were often around a foot or more long also meant they became a very useful protective 'weapon' for any lady that found herself in a difficult or compromising situation. Receiving a purposeful prod from one of these pins was described as being like 'the sting of a hornet' and although I have never been stung by one of these insects, I can imagine it must have been a very painful experience. Such was the size of these pins – excessive in the opinion of some – that they quickly gained notoriety and, in several cities around the world including New York, Hamburg and Berlin, there were proposals to bring in laws to control just how long they could be. Seems like the Health and Safety busybodies were around even then! Their cause in Berlin in particular was bolstered as a result of one nasty accident, reported in a *Daily Mail* article of 17 December 1908 entitled '*Deadly Hatpin – Heavy Casualty List in Berlin*', about one unfortunate lady who, as she rushed into a crowded store to get a sale bargain, walked straight onto the end of one of these pins and was permanently blinded in one eye. Horrific! And in similar vein, the Paris *Daily Mail* in April 1909 reported that a bill was being introduced in the Arkansas legislature in the USA to officially reduce the permitted standard length of these pins to a mere nine inches, and to oblige people take out permits for longer pins. Tram companies in at least one German town also joined in the rumpus and forbade the wearing of these long pins by passengers. Around the world, ever-enterprising individuals spotted an opportunity and patented all sorts of ideas to cap off the sharp end of hatpins to make them safer.

And yet, on a more whimsical note, there were those who found an amusing side to things. Music hall ballads of the later Victorian and Edwardian periods could be pretty bawdy as the composer of the following cockney offering amusingly noted at the time:

Never Go Walking Without Your Hat Pin!

My Granny was a very shrewd old lady,
The smartest woman that I ever met,
She used to say "Now listen to me Sadie,
There's one thing that you never should forget".

Never go walking out without your hat pin.
The law won't let you carry more than that.
For if you go walking out without your hat pin,
You may lose your head as well as lose your hat.

My Granny said men could never be trusted.
No matter how refined they might appear.
She said that many maidens' hearts got busted
Because men never had but one idea.

I've heard that Grandpa really was a mess,
So Grandma knew whereof she spoke I guess.
Never go walking out without your hat pin.
Not even to some very classy joints.
For when a fellow sees you've got a hat pin
He's very much more apt to get the point.

My Mama, too, set quite a bad example.
She never heeded Grandmama's advice.
She found that if you give a man a sample,
The sample somehow never does suffice.

In fact, it's rumoured I might not have been
If Mum had not gone out without her pin.

Never go walking out without your hat pin.
It's about the best protection you have got.
For if you go walking without your hat pin,
You may come home without your you-know-what!

Who's a Pretty Boy Then?

There was one serious (many would say shameful) side effect created by this bourgeoning Edwardian fashion fad however. As you can imagine, with all these feathers on show, it was the international bird population that took a pretty big hit, especially those with bright or distinctive plumage. There seemed to be no end to the 'creative' scope of the milliners with the feathers of herons, egrets (known as 'little snowies'), peacocks, birds of paradise and parrots invariably in their sites and, if you could afford it, you could even have a whole hummingbird! Not to putting too fine a point on it, the future of these specific birds, and indeed many others, was under serious threat. Nothing seemed to be off limits. Use was made of single tail plumes, whole wings from pigeons and other birds, imitation flower and feather sprays (referred to as aigrettes – from the French word for egret) attached to the hat by decorative pins or clips and even, according to a couple of French postcards in my collection entitled 'Mode Chanteclair', what seems to be pretty much a whole chicken! One image which came to light during my research featured almost an entire owl draped around the crown of a hat and another story emerged of an Ipswich lady whose husband banned her from wearing her hat in the countryside during the shooting season. The reason? The lady's hat was festooned with an almost complete pheasant! Just think about it for a moment. Who in their right mind today would walk around with pretty much a whole bird on top of their head?

Feather Farms and Breeders

In the case of ostrich feathers in particular, there were feather farms around the world dedicated to supplying the seemingly unending demands of the millinery and fashion industries. In the early 1900s, probably just about the biggest of these farms was to be found in the Oudtshoorn (pronounced 'Oats–horn') region of Western Cape Province in South Africa, often referred to as 'the Jerusalem of South Africa'. Max Rose, who had arrived in South Africa as an immigrant in 1890 was, by around 1900, the undisputed feather baron in the region. Another successful player in the feather market was Isaac Nurick, whose family had also been immigrants, hailing from the Latvian town of Shavel.

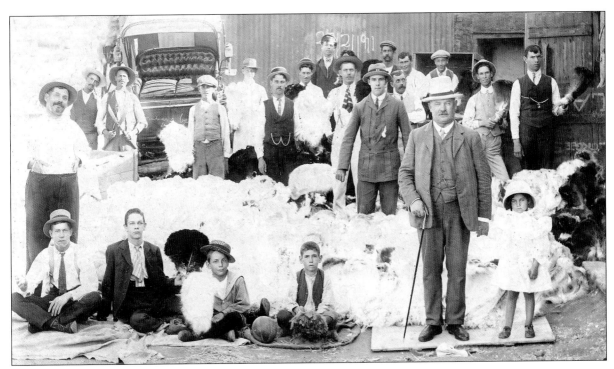

A 1911 picture of the Jewish feather dealer – Mr Isaac Nurick (pictured in the right foreground with the walking stick) and his daughter Ruby, together with around twenty of his staff and a large heap of feathers. Nurick's story is one of rags to riches and back to rags again as he lost everything in a very short space of time when the world ostrich feather industry collapsed almost overnight. *(Image by kind permission of the C.P. Nel Museum, Oudtshoorn, South Africa.)*

The producers in this area, with a certain amount of cross breeding with the Barbary ostrich, produced superb 'double fluff' feathers – at least in the eyes of the milliners and over the late Victorian and early Edwardian periods, the owners had made immense wealth. Back in 1903 it was said that many feathers were fetching $32 per ounce and during 1912, it is claimed that £175 million worth of South African feathers were imported into Britain alone.

In her book, *Plumes: Ostrich Feathers, Jews And A lost World of Global Commerce*, Sarah Abrevaya Stein relates the story of how in 1911, in the search for the best ostriches and thus the best feathers, Russell Thornton, a South African government official, travelled to the Barbary area of North Africa (regions known today as Morocco, Tunisia, Algeria and Libya) with the aim of acquiring breeding pairs of birds to take back to his homeland. Things got a little complicated when no birds were located, but the search continued and some were subsequently located in the Sudan. Moving on to Kano in northern Nigeria – a major trading hub, Thornton and his team got back on track by examining the bales of feathers arriving on incoming Arab caravans. Having ascertained the origins of the good quality feathers, they eventually found what they were after in the French territory of Timbuktu. At this point, they were sanctioned by the South African government to purchase some 150 birds at a cost of £7,000. Then, having been banned by the French authorities from exporting said birds, there followed a cat-and-mouse scenario as the South Africans sought to outwit French 'spies' – which they eventually did. The 'illegal' consignment eventually made its way to the port of Lagos in Nigeria and from there, completed a further 3,000 mile sea journey to Capetown and the ostrich farms of Cape Western Province. Amazingly, some 140 birds survived the trip.

Some of the fortunes made from feathers by the breeders and dealers were translated into very splendid homes, which became known as 'Ostrich Feather Palaces' (see the following section). So sought after were feathers from this area that there was a time when just a single, fairly average, pair of these birds could fetch anything up to £1,000 and the feather industry became a significant part of the South African economy, being fourth only in export value behind diamonds, gold and wool.

An interesting 1907 article from Cape Colony To-day Illustrated by A.E.R. Burton (who gives the impression of not having been to an auction before) offers a very vivid account of the comings and goings at a feather auction of the time. In it he writes:

The conduct of a feather auction is very interesting. There are features about it different to ordinary auctions. For instance, a sale we attended was composed entirely of buyers. The feathers had been entrusted to the auctioneer as broker, and he represented most of the owners. Although the audience was most orderly, it was the keenest gathering imaginable. Jewish buyers in force, with a few slim farmers in opposition, and the cutest auctioneer in command. There were probably £8,000 worth of feathers for sale, so it was a fairly big sale. The first regulation read out was that there should be a reserve price on all feathers, and that they should be sold to the highest bidder above that price. The decision of the auctioneer was always to be final in case of a dispute, and all sales were for spot cash (nobody trusts anybody in the feather business). The attendance at a sale can only be secured by the introduction of an auctioneer and broker, a compound avocation, and from a local bank, and any person, other than the owner or the buyer, who

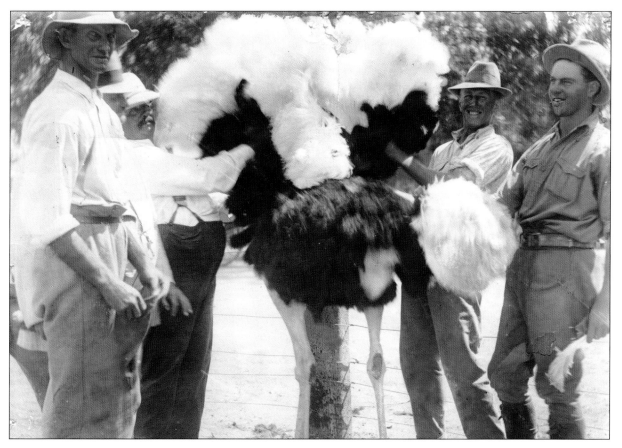

This massive male ostrich was called Cetshwayo – named after the old Zulu king of that name due to his huge size. The bird became famous during the 'Feather Boom' period of 1891 when his owner received an amazing offer of £1,000 for him. This stupendous amount must be compared with the price of a five-seater Ford car in those days, which, according to the *Oudtshoorn Courant* in 1913 cost a full £200. Some bird! Some feathers! (*Image by kind permission of the C.P. Nel Museum, Oudtshoorn, South Africa.*)

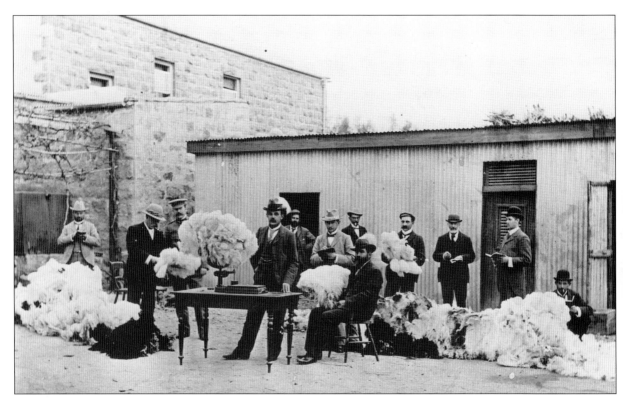

An interesting photograph of feather farmers and dealers busy buying and selling their 'harvest'. The farmers in question were the three Potgieter brothers (pictured in the foreground) and various feather buyers feature at the rear. The man in the uniform is a security guard! £5,000 was made on that particular day. (*Image by kind permission of the C.P. Nel Museum, Oudtshoorn, South Africa.*)

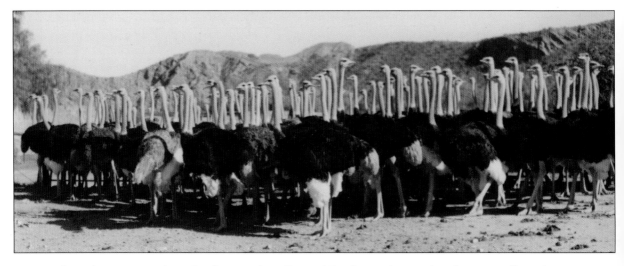

Ostriches on a modern day farm at the village of De Rust where a few farmers still produce beautiful feathers with birds descended from the original bloodline. (*Image by kind permission of the C.P. Nel Museum, Oudtshoorn, South Africa.*)

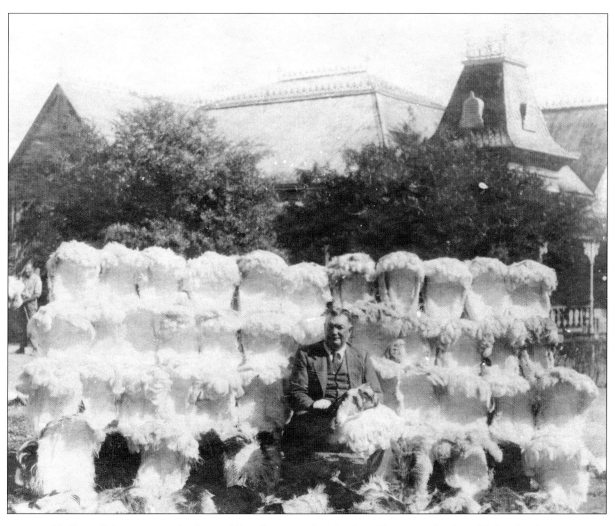

Mr Fanie Schoeman on the farm of Die Denne with a display of his prime feathers. Today, this farm is used as an experimental facility. (*Image by kind permission of the C.P. Nel Museum, Oudtshoorn, South Africa.*)

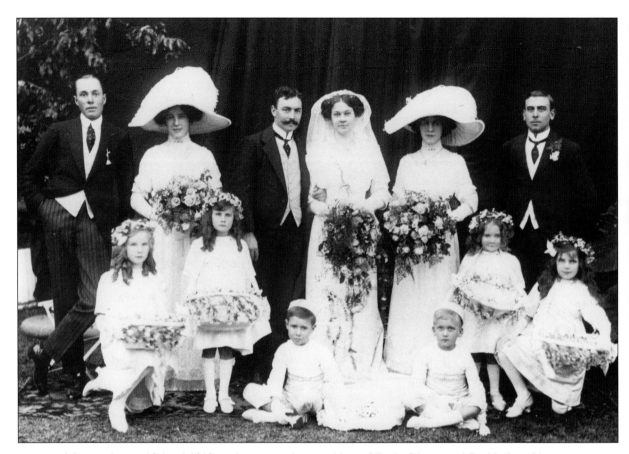

A happy day on 10 April 1912 at the upper class wedding of Emily Olivier and Dr Mathew Heyns. Emily was the daughter of G.C. Olivier – one of the feather barons in the Oudtshoorn area and owner of the 'Towers'. The two bridesmaids with the amazing and elegant feathered hats were Muriel and Annie Foster. (*Image by kind permission of the C.P. Nel Museum, Oudtshoorn, South Africa.*)

wishes to attend must first be properly introduced by the broker or a responsible buyer. There were only three English firms represented.

Most of the feathers in the district are sold out of hand, while they are on the bird – sometimes three months in advance. The broker whose sale we attended informed us that his sales averaged over £60,000 a year. The profits made by individual farmers are enormous. One farmer lately contracted to sell to a local buyer his whole stock of feathers representing the plucking of 2,000 ostriches, at £6 per bird. This was only one of several interests he had. His tenants pay him £3,000 a year. Besides all this he has a large vineyard and orchard, and makes a lot of money out of dried fruit.

However, all 'good' things come to an end as they say and by 1911, with stiff competition from California, the south of France and other locations and the First World War fast approaching, the feather market started to wane. By 1913-14 when, it is estimated, there were around 776,000 ostriches being farmed, and with hostilities about to engulf Europe, the feather market collapsed as hats started to become smaller and less ornate resulting in warehouses around the world being full to the brim with feathers for which there were no buyers. These South African producers, many of whom were either part of, or associated with, the immigrant Russian Lithuanian Jewish community in that neck of the woods and who had been millionaires – or at least very financially well off – one day, suddenly found themselves in much reduced circumstances the next; the bubble, at that time, had just about burst. Isaac Nurick, whom I mentioned previously, lost pretty much everything; leaving his family behind, he 'escaped' to London where he reportedly died penniless. Another story records the reduced circumstances of a particular feather merchant who, in relating the speed with which he had been ruined, detailed how in 1914 he had had a cheque for £100,000 honoured by the local bank but

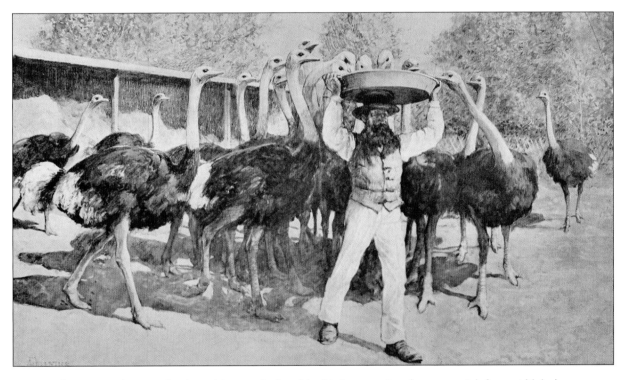

A very novel way to feed ostriches as depicted in this image painted at an ostrich farm at Meknès in Morocco by Anglo French artist – Sir Amédée Forestier 1854 – 1930. Although not originally native to North Africa, one can reasonably assume that, with France's connections to the region, these birds were being reared for their feathers to supply the French millinery trade.

only a year later, a cheque for just £1 had been refused. Dire times; but I bet the ostriches were having a quiet smile! Some reports from the period cynically suggest that certain feather warehouses 'mysteriously' burnt down and received insurance payments – but heaven forbid anything underhand!

A century later, with the world's population having increased many times over, South Africa is still the world's largest producer of ostrich feathers (along with ostrich meat and skin for up market leather goods) although diseases such as bird flu in particular can wreak havoc in an industry which is once again a major contributor to that country's economy. Figures from 2012 show that even though there is no longer a craze for large hats, except perhaps at certain race meetings and the like, there are still around 740 ostrich farms employing over 20,000 people which is quite remarkable. Even a cursory search will astonish the reader at the large number of both wholesalers and retailers around the world still offering these ostrich 'adornments'. But the human race can be very odd and complex and for millennia, certain societies have, for one reason or another, felt the need to decorate themselves with the plumage of assorted colourful birds. For centuries, the traditional 'sing-sing' celebrations of the tribes of the general Borneo and Papua New Guinea regions, Amazonia and the North American Indians were great users of amazing feather bedecked headwear in one ceremonial way or another – but more of this later. In their day, the Edwardian's were not exactly new to the game!

There's an old English saying – mainly associated with the north of the country which goes – 'Where there's muck, there's brass' but in the case of the Oudtshoorn area, maybe that should be changed to 'Where there's feathers, there's brass.'" Crime, it seems, has no limits and in recent times, this part of the world has been plagued by ostrich feather theft. On 10 April 2013, it was announced by the police that five men would appear in court for the alleged theft of ostrich feathers over the previous five months – with an estimated value of R117, 000 (nearly £6,000). The thefts involved the stripping of feathers from numerous live ostriches and in some cases a number of the birds were savagely bludgeoned to death. One of the main targets has been the Western Cape government's research farm at Oudtshoorn. The crime of feather theft has gone on for at least a hundred years – occasioning at one point, the 1907 introduction in South Africa of 'The Ostrich Feather Theft Suppression Bill' but it seems that some things (especially cruelty to our fellow creatures) have not changed that much over the last century.

Ostrich Feather Palaces

Let's face it, the poor old ostrich is not a pretty bird; it's ungainly, can't fly and, as someone once described it, 'one of nature's failed experiments'. Today in South Africa, they are even known somewhat amusingly as 'Karoo sock puppets'. Think about it.

However, as we know, its feathers are really superb and there were those who saw the potential. In the Oudtshoorn area, suddenly a lot of breeders and farmers became very rich and began to look for ways to exhibit their wealth. One of the areas in which they went to town, so to speak, was housing; a goodly number of

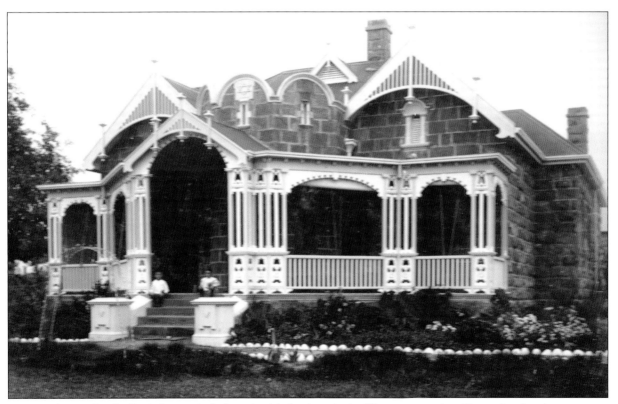

A mansion in Oudtshoorn built by a Jewish feather dealer. The property is still standing but has lost its beautiful verandah and appearance. (*Image by kind permission of the C.P. Nel Museum, Oudtshoorn, South Africa.*)

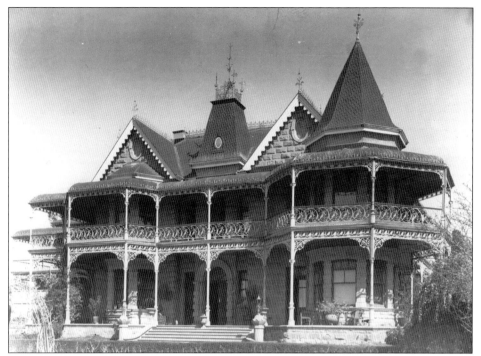

The 'Towers' mansion – built in 1903 by feather baron G.C. Olivier and sadly demolished in 1966 to make way for a school. (*Image by kind permission of the C.P. Nel Museum, Oudtshoorn, South Africa.*)

The wonderfully preserved Mimosa Lodge – originally built for the Jewish feather merchant R. Sladowski. Now owned by the Jonkers family. (*Image by kind permission of the C.P. Nel Museum, Oudtshoorn, South Africa.*)

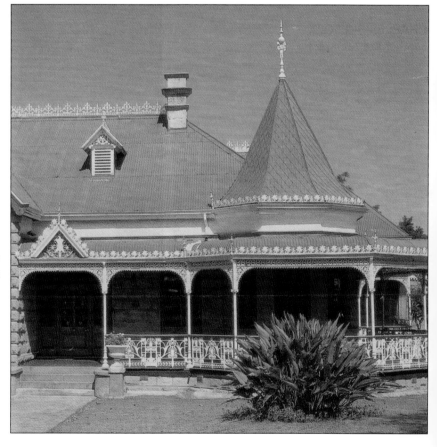

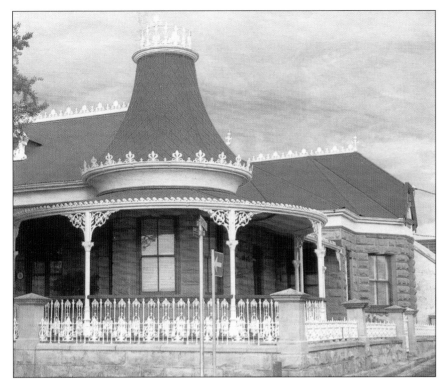

A typical example of one of architect Charles Bullock's ornate 'Feather Palace' homes – designed and built during the Edwardian craze for feathers. (*Image by kind permission of the C.P. Nel Museum, Oudtshoorn, South Africa.*)

them lavished a great deal of money on status symbols and their opulent homes became known as 'Ostrich Feather Palaces'. As can be seen in the preceding images, these were often elaborate affairs which, externally at least and in no way wishing to be rude, have an almost fairytale quality about them. Quite a number of these architecturally remarkable properties still survive to this day in the Oudtshoorn and Little Karoo region of Western Cape Province and offer an insight to the sort of money that was being made from the humble ostrich back in Edwardian times, and the elegant lifestyle that the feather breeders were able to enjoy as a result. Responsible for a number of these 'Palaces' during his six years as a private architect in the area, was Charles Bullock, an English architect who, having arrived in the country in 1890 at the age of 20, must also have done exceedingly well from these elaborate and juicy commissions. Having set up in private practice, Bullock's work on these types of properties began in 1903 with the interiors typically featuring cast iron fireplaces with Art Nouveau tile surrounds, highly decorated ceilings, cornices and dados together with period stained glass. Other architects involved in a number of these types of ornate properties in the area were George Wallace and J.E. Vixeboxes.

Since their original construction and a good deal of renovation work in more recent times, a number of these amazing buildings have been declared National Monuments (and rightly so) with one of them – the magnificent old Boys High School building now housing the superb C.P. Nel Museum.

Parisian Humour

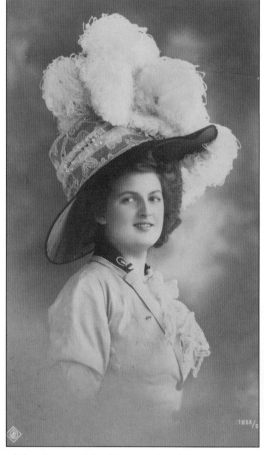

The international thirst for feathers in Edwardian times and the earlier mention of pigeon wings somehow reminds me of the time some years ago when we were hunting for 'Hat' postcards at an early morning street market in a Paris suburb near Saint-Ouen. It was a damp, overcast day and, encountering a stall laden with junk and staffed by a couple of old men, I took the opportunity to try out my schoolboy French. I wished the two old boys 'Bonjour' and enquired 'Avez-vous les cartes postal? Les jollies filles avec grands chapeaux et plumes?' One responded cheerily but the other remained sullenly silent. Had I caused offence? Was my French really that bad? Excusez moi, but the French was actually going OK and, as I was pointing out that the dreary weather was not what we had expected in Paris, a seemingly fearless pigeon suddenly descended at speed from a nearby tree and landed smack in the middle of their stall amongst all the rubbish. Keeping a straight face, I asked 'Combien pour le pigeon?' In an instant, 'Monsieur Sullen', spotting a potential sales opportunity, suddenly came to life and piped up: 'Dix Euros' to which I jokingly responded that the price for the bird was far too high! Sadly, our ageing entrepreneurs had no 'Hat' cards to offer us that day but 'Monsieur Sullen', having suddenly morphed into a deadpan Parisian street comedian eventually saw the funny side and raised a smile. Vive l'humour!

Saving the Birds

Our Victorian and Edwardian forebears, especially the former, had a somewhat peculiar and unenlightened passion for taking birds from the wild. In late Victorian times a House of Commons committee was advised regarding the story of one boy who had captured an amazing 480 goldfinches in just one morning! This type of thoughtless activity together with the subsequent burgeoning trend for feathers and whole birds to be worn on ladies' hats certainly did our avian friends no favours whatsoever. The caged bird trade also continued to be a worrying factor, which persisted on a large scale for many years and this too took its toll on bird populations. Taxidermy was also popular. Look around the contents of any upcoming antique auction and the odds are that you will find a glass case or two filled with an assortment of colourful stuffed birds.

A period of ten years or more – 'the Age of Extermination' as it has been referred to by historians – saw the slaughter, carnage and shockingly inhumane actions of the feather hunters, one of whom in the UK was said to have taken over 4,000 birds in just one year, is illustrated by the fact that sometimes the wings of birds, particularly gulls and kittiwakes, were simply ripped off whilst the birds were still alive and what was left of the hapless creature was simply thrown back into the sea.

But this slaughter was not new. In an essay in 2000, R.J. Moore-Colyer, refers back to the situation in the 1860s and details –

As London and provincial dealers offered one shilling each for the wings of "white gulls"... excursion trains left London for locations as far apart as Flamborough Head and the Isle of White carrying beer-swilling plumage hunters and their rook rifles towards the killing grounds.

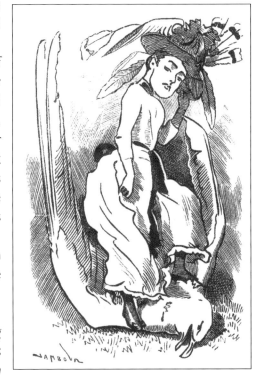

A rather macabre cartoon of the period drawing the association between the use of bird feathers on large hats and the destruction of birds which took place to get them.

Even back in 1887 in the 17 September edition of the topical magazine *Punch*, a poem – author unknown, entitled 'A PLEA FOR THE BIRDS' (To the Ladies of England) floridly outlined the problem and concern.

It reads:

Lo! the sea-gulls slowly whirling
Over all the silver sea,
Where the white-toothed waves are curling,
And the winds are blowing free.
There's a sound of wild commotion,
And the surge is stained with red;
Blood incarnadines the ocean,
Sweeping round old Flamborough Head.

For the butchers come unheeding
All the torture as they slay,
Helpless birds left slowly bleeding,
When the wings are reft away.
There the parent bird is dying,
With the crimson on her breast,
While her little ones are lying
Left to starve in yonder nest.

What dooms all these birds to perish,
What sends forth these men to kill,
Who can have the hearts that cherish
Such designs of doing ill?
Sad the answer: English ladies
Send those men, to gain each day
What for matron and for maid is
All the Fashion, so folks say.

Feathers deck the hat and bonnet.
Though the plumage seemeth fair,
Punch, whene'er he looks upon it,
Sees that slaughter in the air.
Many a fashion gives employment
Unto thousands needing bread,
This, to add to your enjoyment,
Means the dying and the dead.

Wear the hat, then, sans the feather,
English women, kind and true;
Birds enjoy the summer weather
And the sea as much as you.
There's the riband, silk, or jewel,
Fashion's whims are oft absurd;
This is execrably cruel;
Leave his feathers to the bird!

Seriously nasty stuff this and indeed, such was the rate of 'kill' or capture in those days that questions were raised in parliament at one point. The Royal Society for the Protection of Birds (which was originally founded in Didsbury, Manchester in 1889 by Emily Williamson, wife of the explorer Robert Wood Williamson, and known in its infancy as 'The Plumage League') was invariably to the fore in campaigning against the use of feathers, as was Eliza Phillips, one of their most prominent members. Having been awarded its Royal Charter in 1904 the RSPB, as it's commonly known today, soon gained a number of influential members including the Ranee of Sarawak and the Dutchess of Portland who was to become the Society's first president. The RSPB initially concerned itself with two basic tenets:

1) That Members shall discourage the wanton destruction of Birds and interest themselves with their protection.

2) That Lady-Members shall refrain from wearing feathers from any bird not killed for the purposes of food – the ostrich only excepted.

In 1908 there was also an attempt to get the Importation of Plumage (Prohibition) Bill through the House of Commons but it failed to get passed first time round and that particular victory was only achieved some thirteen years later in 1921 – some three years after the end of the First World War when the fashion for large hats smothered with feathers had all but waned anyway. Still, better late than never. In reality, the law didn't actually come into full force until April 1922.

Despite the RSPB's earlier successes in the late Victorian years, the feather trade, aided and abetted by the Edwardians, continued apace. As an example of the sheer scale, it was reported that in 1911, over 41,000 humming bird skins were sold in London alone. To counter the growing concern, the feather suppliers would often claim that the feathers they were providing were shed naturally by the birds but in almost all cases, this was absurdly untrue.

Even Queen Alexandra banned ladies from Court if they were wearing osprey

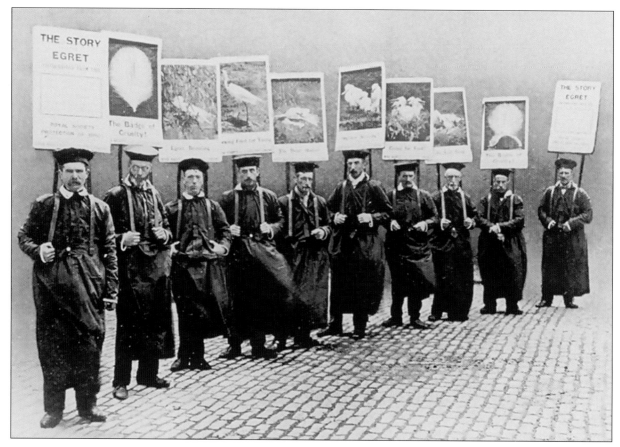

In July 1911, a group of RSPB supporters (in rather strange outfits) with placards/sandwich boards, marching in London in protest against the use of Egret feathers on hats. (*Image by kind permission of The Royal Society for the Protection of Birds.*)

feathers on their hats, although it seems like the poor old ostrich, receiving no specific protection, had got the Royal 'thumbs down' and drawn the short straw (or should I say the short feather) once again. Ostriches it seems were of somewhat less value than ospreys in bird society.

In 1906 at the Annual General Meeting of the RSPB, Royal support was evident in a letter from the queen herself in which she stated that she 'never wears Egret plumes herself and will certainly do all in her power to discourage the cruelty practiced

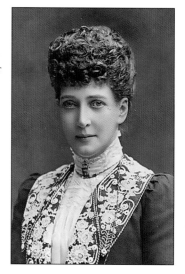

In their earlier days, the RSPB were more than pleased to have the support of Queen Alexandra in their fight against the use of feathers and the huge destruction of the bird population.

on these beautiful birds' further offering the president of the Society – the Duchess of Portland full permission to use her name – 'in any way you think best to conduce to the protection of birds'.

Similarly, in America, partly as the result of the growing unease of enlightened people such as the Boston socialites Harriet Hemenway and her cousin Mina Hall, the Audubon Society was formed in 1905, dedicated to the memory of French/American John James Audubon (1785–1851). A truly talented man and probably best remembered today for his magnificently illustrated book: *The Birds of America*. Audubon, who led an amazing life one way or another, was a highly respected ornithologist and naturalist, and arguably one of the very best bird illustrators that ever lived. But, some fifty years after his passing, as the war on birds continued apace, the Audubon Society, grew in stature and continually voiced its concern as many colourful birds both in that country and around the world were 'harvested' to the brink of extinction or at least very serious depletion.

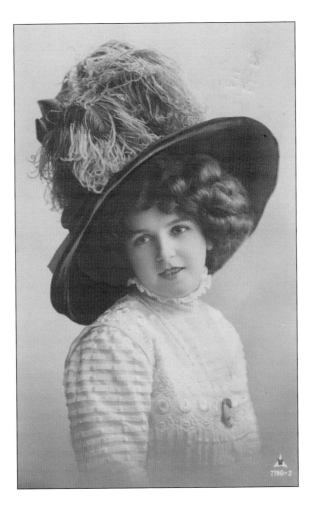

Absolute Butchery

Butchery of birds for either food or feathers is no new thing as the 1598 image of Dutch explorers killing parrots in Mauritius depicts. By the Edwardian era however, some 400 years or so later, it had become just about as bad as it could get. In 1908, the British government outlawed the commercial hunting of birds of paradise in the parts of New Guinea under their rule but sadly, it took the Dutch

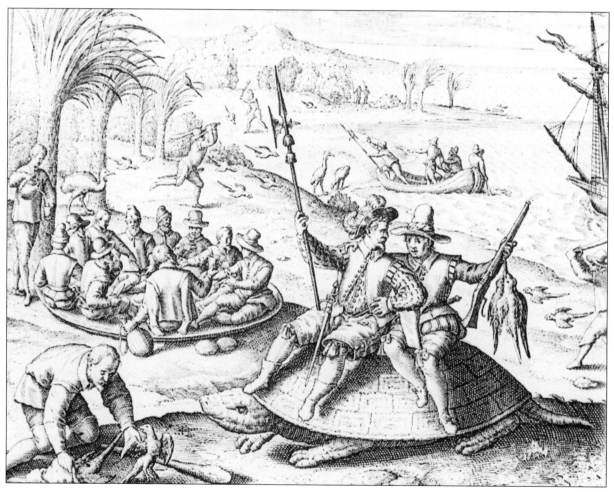

Dutch explorers on Mauritius featured in this 1598 image, wreaking havoc on the local parrot population.

authorities another twenty-three years to follow suit in their own Dutch New Guinea.

During the Victorian and Edwardian eras, birds of paradise paid the price for simply being what they were – colourful and attractive. Today, through the media, television and various wildlife programmes, we know them for what they are – beautiful and amazing creatures. But for several hundred years, these birds had been something of a mystery and the only known information about them came from the relatively few dried corpses and skins that made their way back to Europe. They had been spotted in wonderment by Magellan's men several hundred years earlier in 1522 and although three skins (it is said) came back with them aboard the ship 'Victoria', little fact about these birds was known.

That started to change in 1854 when the naturalist Alfred Russell Wallace visited New Guinea to study them followed in 1876 by the Italian Luigi D'Albertis who, in his double volume account of his expeditions, related several brushes with curious natives. Thus, by the end of the nineteenth century, people were starting to become much more aware of these birds, especially those within millinery trade who saw their gorgeous feathers as money-making additions to their hat creations. The chase was on and, before more enlightened views held sway and society came to its senses, there was only going to be one winner with the poor old New Guinea birds of paradise – particularly the Greater Bird of Paradise, with its colourful tail feathers – very much on the losing side. All that carnage, just to satisfy the whims of fashion. The habits, lives, conservation and beauty of these birds were of no consequence to the hunters, and the odd surviving examples of Edwardian feather-covered hats on display in museums around the world today offer mute examples of what was really going on.

Grandiose names for the many varieties of birds of paradise were often the order of the day. Those that 'christened' them seemed to have taken the view that they should be named after various dignitaries and Royals of the period and we thus have the likes of Princess Stephanie's bird of paradise, Count Raggi's, Victoria's Rifle bird, Prince Rudolf's, Emperor and The King of Saxony etc. Between the years of 1905–1920, the export of their skins to the auction houses of London, Amsterdam and Paris was estimated to be between 30,000 and 80,000 per year with hunters from China, Malaya and Australia (to name just three) moving in to make their fortunes.

In New Guinea, described by some as 'the land that time forgot', the rain forest territory of the Yonggom people between the rivers Ok Tedi and Muyu was a popular and prolific hunting ground with the locals often using feathers as currency. In the ensuing years, and having established at least a modicum of rapport with the locals in terms of trading, peoples like the Yonggom would readily supply the birds of paradise in return for such things as axes, knives and other European 'goodies'.

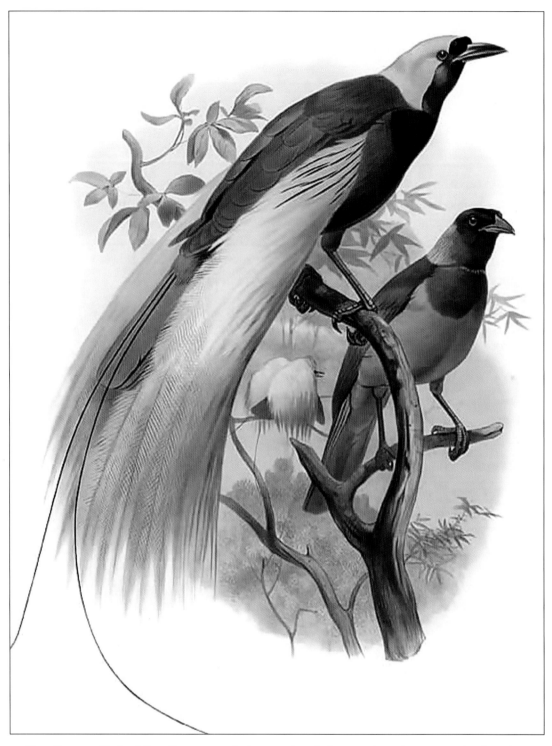

The Greater Bird of Paradise – a typical example of the amazing plumage to be found on numerous birds of paradise. Easy to see why the Edwardian milliners loved them for their colour and decorative value.

The hunting season usually ran from April until September and the Yonggom knew that, during this period, mature birds would assemble in large numbers to display. Engrossed in their courtship displays, the birds were thus easy prey for the hunters who took full advantage. (For those with an interest in this particular field, there is a very interesting article from the Penn Museum by Stuart Kirsch, which covers the subject in much more detail.)

But it was not only in the rainforests of New Guinea that the destruction of birds for their feathers was so savage, and it would take a very perverse point a view to describe it in any other way. For the hunters in Florida's Everglades in America there were no 'closed' seasons. The plumage hunters wrought utter havoc, many often resorting to the use of the almost noiseless rifles or small calibre guns to do their dirty work. As ornithologist William Earle Dodge Scott – curator of the Museum of Biology at Princeton, put it: 'The almost noiseless Flobert rifle … whose report is hardly louder than the snapping of a twig.'

In another 1887 report by the ornithologist William Earle Dodge Scott, curator of the Princeton museum of biology and made bird collecting forays to Florida, he gives details of a scene of horrific slaughter which to came across.

The trees were full of nests, some of which still contained eggs, and hundreds of broken eggs strewed the ground everywhere. Fish Crows and both kinds of Buzzards were present in great numbers and were rapidly destroying the remaining eggs. I found a huge pile of dead, half decayed birds lying on the ground, which had apparently been killed for a day or two. All of them had the 'plumes' taken with a patch of skin from the back, and had the wings cut off; otherwise they were uninjured. I counted over two hundred birds treated in this way … I do not know of a more horrible and brutal exhibition of wanton destruction than that which I witnessed here.

The colourful Carolina Parakeet was just one of numerous breeds to suffer terribly. Apart from obtaining its feathers, it was considered an agricultural pest and was slaughtered in huge numbers. Forest clearance, which had started in earnest in the 1800's did nothing to help its cause. And so after around 1860 it was little seen or reported and was deemed to be extinct by the 1920s. The plight of the shore birds of that area fared little better being reduced to just five per cent of their original numbers in a relatively short space of time. Egret feathers in particular were also popular, particularly those that were referred to as 'nuptial plumes', which were grown by the birds for courtship purposes each year. The fact that, unlike some birds, both the females as well as the males were blessed with beautiful feathers, meant that invariably both adults were killed for their plumes leaving the young both parentless and defenceless to die a lingering death. (One section of the popular Sears catalogue in 1911 even shows a whole page entirely devoted to bird wings which are described as 'Bargains in Imported Trimming Wings' – on offer from thirty or forty cents to a dollar or two).

On this subject, ornithologist and conservationist T. Gilbert Pearson recalled:

> A few miles north of Waldo, our party came upon a little swamp where we had been told herons bred in numbers. Upon approaching the place the screams of young birds reached our ears. The cause of this soon became apparent by the buzzing of green flies and heaps of dead Herons festering in the sun, with the back of each bird raw and bleeding … Young herons had been left by the scores in the nests to perish from exposure and starvation.

The American Ornithologists Union, founded in 1883 and similar to its British counterpart (founded in 1858) referred to: 'Women as a Bird Enemy'. On another occasion in 1886, the growing danger to numerous bird species had been overtly illustrated to Frank Chapman of the American Museum of Natural History in New York as he walked through Manhattan on a couple of occasions – spotting the feathers of forty-two different native species on 542 passing ladies' hats. Although it took a further twenty years or so, the New York State Audubon Plumage Law was enacted in 1910, which banned the sales of feathers from native birds and the importation of 'aigrettes' and other feathers. Previous to this, the Lacey Act of 1900 had helped the situation to a degree, as did the Migratory Birds Treaty Act in 1918. Nevertheless, in spite of the objections, and with feathers having risen from $32 per ounce to $80 per ounce by 1903, the trend seemed unstoppable.

The Lacey Act of 1900 had bolstered existing laws in that it prohibited interstate trade in wildlife and wildlife products (in this case feathers) protected by state legislation. Numerous states had protected their own native birds from the feather hunters who, in response, strove to get around the law by transporting their ill-gotten gains to states where the birds were not regarded as native, and sell them there. If they were caught and found guilty, both the seller and receiver would be hit with cripplingly onerous fines.

One of the first and more notable violations of the Act took place in 1909 and was perpetrated on Laysan – a tiny island in the Pacific some 808 nautical miles north-west of Honalulu in Hawaii. A German immigrant and feather merchant cum entrepreneur by the name of Max Schlemmer – often known as the 'King of Laysan' (and at other times 'Schlemmer the Slaughterer') hired twenty-three Japanese labourers to slaughter over 300,000 slow moving and clumsy Laysan and Black-

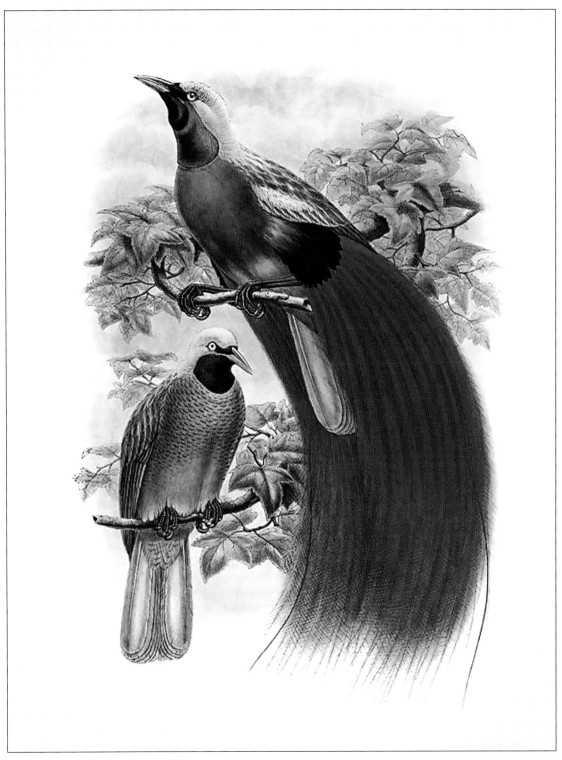

Fabulous red plumes – a ready target for the feather dealers, fashion houses and milliners of Europe.

footed Albatrosses which were nesting on the island. Absolutely no mercy was shown and many simply had their wings hacked off and were left to die, while numerous others were simply herded into a nearby cistern and left to starve to death. Discovering what was going on, a zoology professor from the College of Honalulu informed the US authorities (Layson being part of US territory) whereupon the Secretary of the Navy immediately dispatched a revenue cutter (the Thetis) to the island, there to find carcasses, bones and three large containers of wings, feathers and skins. Utterly unforgivable.

The guilty parties were immediately arrested and sent for trial in Honalulu. Later that same year, President Theodore Roosevelt was prompted to issue an Executive order creating the Hawiian Islands an official reservation for birds.

Gradually, at least some feather hunters saw the error of their ways. In his book *Everglades Lawman: True Stories of Game Wardens in the Glades* published by the Pineapple Press, James Huffstodt relates:

> *The plume hunters left devastation and the stench of decay in their wake. Even some hardened shooters were soon sickened by the brutal execution. One plume hunter, who would later quit the bloody trade, was consumed by guilt as he surveyed the hideous aftermath of an hour's work. 'The heads and necks of the young birds were hanging out of the nests by the hundreds' he wrote. 'I am done with bird hunting forever'.*

A Damascene conversion if ever there was one!

Not everybody in high places was against the feather trade however, and numerous politicians spoke out against the reduction – citing the loss of jobs and employment. During the course of a debate on the Tariff Bill in 1913, a certain, (seemingly uncaring) American Senator by the name of Reed said:

> *I really want to know why there should be any sympathy or sentiment about a long-legged, long-beaked, long-necked bird that lives in the swamps and eats tadpoles and fish and crawfish and things of that kind; why we should worry ourselves into a frenzy because some lady adorns herself with one of its feathers, which appears to be the only use it has.*

And that has to be just about as callous and unenlightened as anybody can get.

On another occasion, the outcry against the slaughter of birds for millinery purposes by the American public was countered as being ridiculous by the publication *Milliner and Dressmaker* which, in its wisdom, cautioned that 'the result of

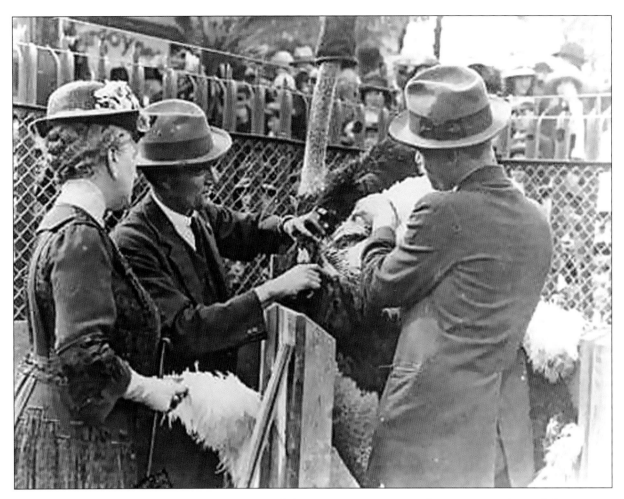

Although the Edwardian period had passed, this more recent picture shows two members of the South African feather industry in action at the 1924/25 British Empire Wembley Exhibition. The lady on the left is almost certainly Queen Alexandra (who died in that same year) observing the clipping of ostrich wing feathers with the bird secured in a 'plucking box'. This demonstration was pretty certainly set up in an effort counter anti-feather campaigners such as the RSPB and to show that the process didn't harm the birds in any way when the feathers were 'harvested'. Note how the ostrich has a bag over its head. *(Image by kind permission of the C.P. Nel Museum, Oudtshoorn, South Africa.)*

any ban on the use of feathers would be to deprive hundreds of respectable young women of their livelihood in the trade.' So that makes it OK then?

In the UK, fairly similar sentiments were raised by a certain Lieutenant Colonel Archer-Shee, a London member of Parliament, who, when speaking in the Commons against the Plumage Bill of 1920, noted that many of his fellow MPs had themselves arrived at the chamber clad from head to toe in animal products such as fleeces of sheep, shoes made of cattle hide, rabbit-skin hats and with some even sporting the odd mink coat. What about the cruelty involved in obtaining those particular materials he pondered? Surely, the killing a 'few' birds to satisfy female fashion was but a drop in the ocean of cruelty? Other members expressed sentiments along the same lines.

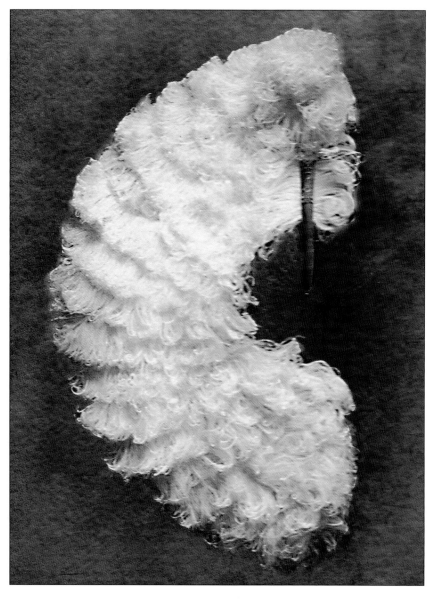

An ostrich feather fan presented to Her Majesty Queen Alexandra at the opening of the Cape Exhibition in London 1907. (*Image by kind permission of the C.P. Nel Museum, Oudtshoon, South Africa.*)

Plumassiers

Unsurprisingly, this burgeoning fashion fad led to workshops springing up all around the world where feathers were laboriously prepared for the millinery trade by groups of specialists called 'Plumassiers'. Literally translated from the French, this word means 'feather workers'.

An entry in the 1901 edition of *The Encyclopaedia Britannica* describes the term thus: 'The art of the plumassier embraces the cleaning, bleaching, dying, curling and making up of ostrich and other plumes and feathers'.

And it was reckoned by some that during the 'working' lifespan of an single ostrich, which was relieved of its feathers every eight or nine months, around a total of 300 plumes could be 'harvested' from the unfortunate creature. Whilst London was recognised as the world auction centre of the plumage trade with companies such as Hale and Sons, Dalton & Young and Figgis & Co to the fore, Paris and New York in turn were the main manufacturing centres. Paris in particular had an extraordinary number of 'Plumassiers' and New York's Lower East Side had many feather 'sweatshops'. It was not uncommon for tuberculosis, bad skin and even fever to be rife among the workers due to the dust and fluff floating around in these dark, cluttered and low paying establishments – a high price to pay in health terms for the 'fashion' of others.

The equally degrading image of little boys climbing up the inside of chimneys in days gone by readily comes to mind. Payment for such demeaning work as 'Willowing' was also systematically cut to the bone by unscrupulous employers. ('Willowing' can best be described in modern day terms as roughly equating to hair extensions but using feathers as opposed to hair). A poem of the period taken from *Sorrowful Rhymes of Working Children in 1911* illustrates the point:

> *How doth the manufacturer*
> *Improve the ostrich tail?*
> *By willowing the scraggy ends*
> *Until they're fit for sale*
> *How cheerfully he sits and smiles*
> *Throughout the livelong day*
> *While children knot the tiny flues*
> *And make the plumes that pay.*

But desperate people, living seemingly hopeless lives, will do desperate things to survive and make a little money. The New York labour laws sought to combat the use of dirt poor 'home worker' children and poverty stricken immigrants within the feather industry (amongst others) but the sheer numbers involved, and a shortage of officers to enforce the law, meant it was, by and large, a losing battle. These often hellish conditions in New York in locations such as Division St. on Manhattan's Lower East Side are further illustrated by a range of sombre pictures taken by the American sociologist and photographer Lewis W Hine – well known for his work among the poor and under privileged in the lower reaches of American society. It was estimated that there were around 83,000 people involved in the feather industry across America during the early years of the twentieth century; for those who might be interested, a selection of Hine's images of grim New York feather workshops, illustrating the

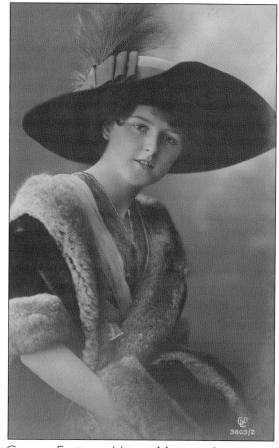

hellish working conditions, is to be found in the George Eastman House Museum in Rochester, New York State. Having said all this, it has to be very difficult for us today, with our relatively comfortable lives, to truly imagine the reality of life for these struggling feather workers. One is forced to ask oneself whether the upmarket ladies of the day around the world, in their spectacular hats, had the slightest idea – or ever spared a moment's thought for – all the folk who made their finery possible. In many cases, probably not.

The Feather King

Another interesting story concerning the feather industry in New York details a 'gentleman' by the name of Isidor Cohnfeld —subsequently known as 'the Feather King' whose word became law in the feather trade. Cohnfeld, originally a penniless immigrant from Germany, was responsible in 1886 for the construction on the corner of Bleecker and Greene Streets in Manhattan of what was to become known as the Cohnfeld Building, where he employed hundreds of young women in the bleaching, dying, sewing and trimming of feathers. The *New York Times* called it 'The finest feather factory in the world'. Only one year later in 1887 however, Cohnfeld, mortgaged up to the hilt and finding himself in serious financial trouble, apparently did a runner to Canada – with more than $250,000 in his suitcase. His factory became known as 'Cohnfeld's Folly'! The *New York Times* who, just twelve months previously, had been singing his praises, now referred to him as 'the ostrich feather plunger!' and just to add insult to injury, the Cohnfeld Building burned down in 1891.

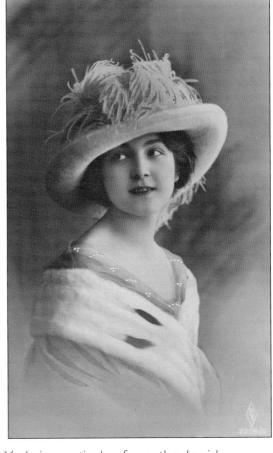

Meanwhile, on New York's Lower East Side, the feather company of Lowenstein and Gray had serious, on-going problems with workers (many of whom were of Russian Jewish descent) striking over wages and conditions. An excellent book on the subject of the world feather industry in general, and New York in particular, from the Jewish perspective is *Plumes* by Sarah Stein (Yale University Press).

Monsieur Methot

Yet another of the numerous New York plumassiers was a Frenchman called H. Method who operated his business from 29 West 34th Street under the trading name of 'French Feather Dyer and Dresser'. Method tempted potential customers with a sort of 'drop in' service by offering 'Feathers Curled on Your Hat While You Wait' and 'Willow and French Plumes also Handsome Paris Novelties made from fine old Discarded Feathers – YOU WILL BE SURPRISED WITH THE RESULT.'

Method determinedly advertised that 'The Dying and Curling of Plumes takes its place as one of the FINE ARTS.'

He also goes on to say that: 'Bleaching and Cleansing have long been a Scientific Speciality with us – delicate operations, which require the most care. With the Method facilities, the cost is very slight and the work quickly done.'

He further points out that You will be surprised at the possibilities of old pieces. They serve in rebuilding the most elaborate plumes at half the cost.

As an early sort of 'mail order' service he requests that the customer 'Send two-cent stamp for our special mailing envelope in which you send your feathers to us and we will gladly advise you as to the best manner of remodelling them. Seems like Monsieur Method was something of a lateral thinker with his eye on the half chance.

An advertisement in the programme of Boston's Plymouth Theatre in 1913 shows us that Method was by then also providing his services in that city from 59 Temple Place, Blake Building, Elevator – 'Sign of the Golden Ostrich.' Had he moved out of New York to the slightly more genteel Boston or was this just another branch that he had set up as part of his business expansion?

At any rate, he was offering: 'Ostrich Feathers Dyed, Cleaned or Curled – Willow Plumes Cleaned or Dyed Successfully.

He also states that:

Your old feathers can be made into beautiful French Plumes by the small addition of new tops, or any of the 1912 novelties at small cost.

The fact that we are the pioneer firm in Boston specializing in OSTRICH FEATHER WORK, having been in business for over 33 years, assures you better work and lower prices than elsewhere.

We would like to advise you about your feather work for the Fall. Samples shown for the latest Ostrich Novelties. Why not inspect our fall line of Ostrich Feathers.

Canada's 'Greatest Store'

Fashion it seems has pretty much no bounds whatever era you may live in and bumper sized, feather covered hats had seamlessly spread around the world during Edward VII's reign. For students of Edwardian fashion today, it is worth researching T. Eaton Co Limited of Toronto in Canada.

Established in 1869, it was, by 1896, billing itself as 'Canada's Greatest Store' and was obviously a very switched on operator in the retail world. Eaton's produced many product catalogues – the first being in 1884, and some expanding to several hundred pages over the years. As part of their range, they offered a large choice of assorted fashion products, which were often referred to as 'The Edwardian Look'. Maybe the Canadian tastes were a little more conservative than those of their European cousins however; hats from London and Paris were often expensive to import and the French designs often being considered a touch outré. Eaton's got over this to some degree by having its own millinery department claiming to employ several hundred young women, most of whom would have been earning no more than $20 per month. This claim is partially supported by photographs from 1902 and 1904 from the Archives of Ontario; their workroom appear packed with young ladies beavering away producing vast quantities of hats 'to suit the taste and style of Canadians'. Further interesting reference to the company's millinery operation may be found in the form of a number of stereoscopic images held at the National Gallery of Canada and dating from around 1906 onwards.

The company also offered to the millinery trade (and those customers who wanted to 'do their own thing') a range of untrimmed hats together with trimming supplies such as feathers. A search through the company's archive catalogues will yield many interesting visual examples of ladies outfits – and hats in particular, smothered with copious quantities of feathers on page after page.

Maison Lemarié

In mainland Europe, it was estimated that by 1919 in the French capital alone there were around 425 'feather establishments' serving the fashion industry with probably the best known being the legendary and creative Maison Lemarié. Today, that figure is said to be down to just one or two and whilst Maison Lemarié, founded in 1880 by Palmyra Coyette under the business description of 'studio of plumes-for-garments' still survives, having been acquired by Chanel in 1996, many colourful and exotic birds around the world must be feeling just a little happier these days! Having said that, the house of Maison LeMarie, (which incidentally still has a very comprehensive period feather archive acquired over the years when various competitors were bought out or ceased to trade. Many of the feathers are from birds which are protected species today), continues to produce superb millinery and associated haute couture items that include the use of legal, non-restricted feathers from South Africa such as vultures, swans, peacocks and, of course, the perennially farmed ostrich. High-end clients of Maison LeMarie today, apart of course from its owner Chanel, include Givenchy, Dior and Lacroix in France, and Dolce & Gabanna, Valentino and Armani in Italy.

Let us not forget the Parisian courtesans – great patrons of the fashion world in their day. They had to look good for the class of client they were after and for those ladies of easy virtue who had made it to the top so to speak, 'Les Grandes Horizontals' as they were known, money for fashion was not in short supply. Three of the most famous – 'Les Grandes Trois', – Emilienne d'Alençon, the beautiful Liane de Pougy and Caroline Otero (La Belle Otero) could often be seen in the vicinity of the Bois de Boulogne and other fashionable spots sporting, at times, large feather bedecked hats as they went about their business cementing their 'social' contacts.

The Amazing Coco Chanel

There can be few people in the western world and further afield who are not familiar with the name of Coco Chanel. Her amazing life and times have long been well documented by researchers and authors over the years, but in terms of her involvement with the creation and development of large hats in the earlier part of her career (during the Edwardian era), I felt that a brief summary of her outstanding contribution to the world of fashion well worth inclusion in this book.

The story of Gabrielle Chanel (as she was known at birth) is very much the classic 'rags to riches' scenario and she is the only fashion designer to gain a listing in *Time Magazine*'s top 100 most influential people of the twentieth century. One can find many references to Chanel's middle name being listed as 'Bonheur' but company authorities inform me that this name did not actually appear on her birth certificate.

From a tough start in life, Gabrielle or Coco as she became known, was determined, ambitious and energetic in all she did. She became a prolific designer and her legacy today is reflected not only in haute couture clothing fashions (who is not familiar with 'the little black dress' and the Chanel suit?), but also across a wide range of upmarket jewellery, bags, perfumes, Suntan lotion and many associated products. Once established, Chanel was arguably the leading icon of fashion in the twentieth century.

The profusion of stories surrounding Chanel during her colourful life is, seemingly endless – featuring associations with the well-connected and wealthy, high profile affairs and the apocryphal story that she gained the name Coco as a result of the fabulous parties she threw in Paris where cocaine was an integral part of the menu. Quite a gal and a tough 'cookie!'

But to revert to Chanel's beginnings: she was born out of wedlock in August 1883 to laundrywoman Eugenie Jeanne Devolle and Albert Chanel in the Sisters of Provence charity hospital in Saumur, France. The couple were subsequently married in the following year and the young Gabrielle was raised, along with her four siblings, in a one-room lodgings in the small town of Brive la Gaillarde. There, her father Albert operated as an itinerant and low-income street vendor – peddling work clothes and undergarments. So far so bad!

When her mother died in 1895, the 12-year-old Coco and her two sisters were sent by their father to the convent of Aubazine in the Correze region of central France. The religious order there – The Congregation of the Sacred Heart was 'founded to care for the poor and rejected, including running homes for abandoned and orphaned girls.' After such a poor start in life, who would have guessed, what the years to come would bring to the latent designer?

After some six years at Aubazine, Coco had learned the art of sewing and gained employment as a seamstress. But when not plying her trade with the needle, she sang in cabaret, made her stage debut and subsequently performed at various venues frequented by the military – especially in the town of Moulins. Her youthful charms caught the eye of many but her singing voice was not up to par and her hoped-for stage career did not materialize.

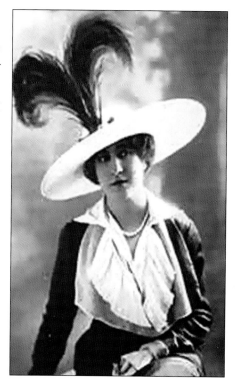

Chanel's friend – the French actress Gabrielle Dorziat modelling one of the former's early hat creations as featured in *Les Modes* magazine in May 1912.

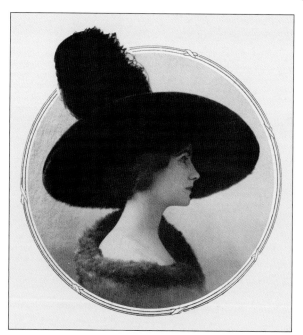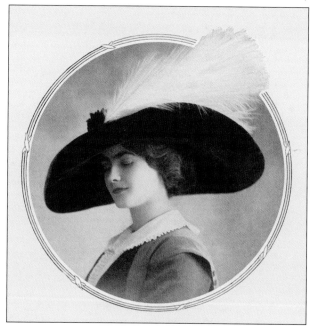

Early images of Coco Chanel wearing examples of her own feathered hat creations. (*Comoedia Illustré 1910 Photo Félix/All Rights Reserved.*)

152

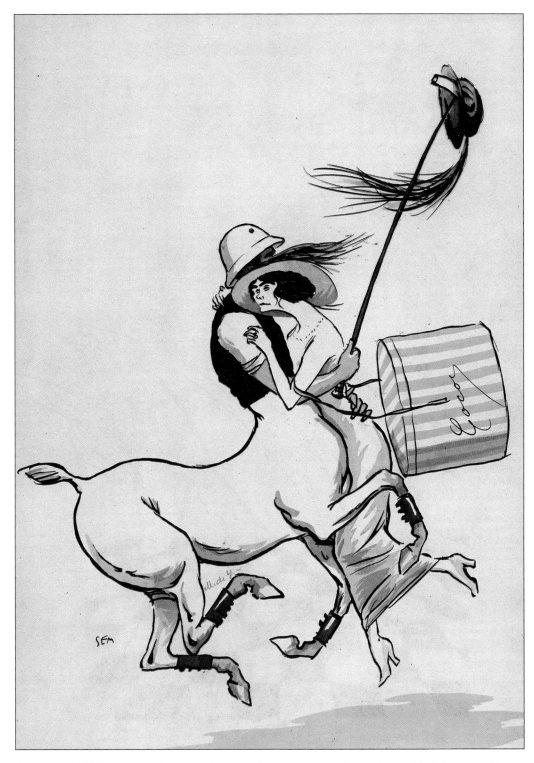

An original 1913 caricature by artist Georges Goursat Sem – 'Tangoville sur Mer' featuring Chanel dancing with her polo playing lover Arthur 'Boy' Capel. (*Image by kind permission of Chanel, Paris.*)

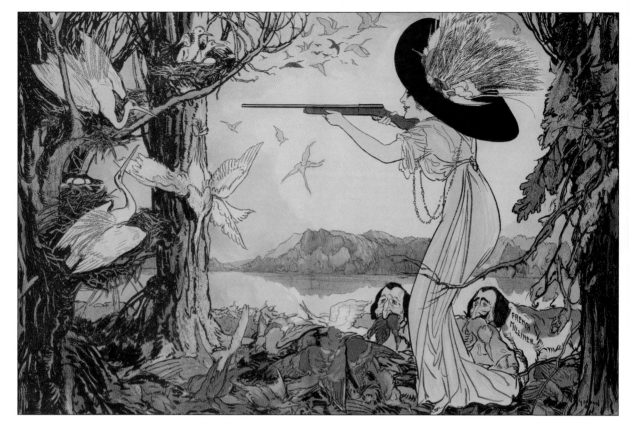

It has been suggested that this illustration of a fashionable lady in her large, feather bedecked hat, shooting exotic birds – by the Scottish artist Gordon Ross – 1873–1946, (originally featured in *PUCK* magazine in May 1911), was very probably 'aimed' at Coco Chanel as a form of protest against the use of feathers on her early millinery. (Note the heap of dead birds at her feet and the two nearby dogs, one of whom is labelled 'French Milliner.')

During this period, Chanel became the mistress of the wealthy textile heir Etienne Balsan, and for the next three years lived a self-indulgent lifestyle while cultivating the wealthy social set who revelled in their fortunes and decadent gratification. You can almost see Chanel's future starting to map itself out.

In 1908 Chanel began a second affair, which lasted nine years, with a friend of Balsan – the never faithful polo playing Captain Arthur Edward 'Boy' Capel During this time Chanel began designing hats – an venture which evolved into a commercial enterprise. She gained her licence as a milliner in 1910 and opened a boutique (supposedly financed by Capel) at 21 rue Cambon in Paris, under the name Chanel Modes, from where she designed and sold her outsized millinery creations. Many of these featured copious quantities of feathers which were often referred to as 'birds nests'.

It was at this time that Chanel's millinery career really took off when the renowned theatre actress Gabrielle Dorziat wore her Edwardian style hats in Fernand Nozière's play Bel Ami in 1912 and later in the same year in the publication Les Modes. Coco was on her way and her large feathered hats, to a considerable degree, had opened the door to what became an astounding and diverse life that most of us can only dream about. Merci Coco pour les modes.

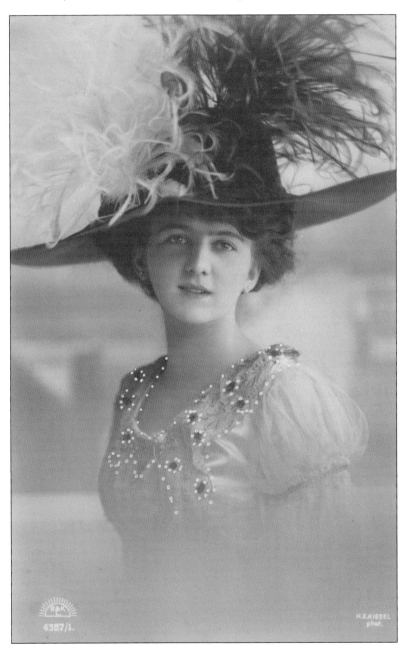

Paranoia?

In my early days of postcard collecting, it felt to me as though hardened card enthusiasts seemed to look down on my 'wants'. After all, who would be interested in this bottom of the market fancy hat stuff? Perhaps I was becoming a touch paranoid, but at postcard fairs I always seemed to get the impression that heads were turning in disdain and did I detect the odd knowing smile from other nearby collectors when they heard me ask the dealers for 'Any Photographic Glamour?' Likewise, it was not at all unusual for the odd dealer to hand me a bunch of nudes! In response I would pass them back immediately and say something like: For heaven's sake, I was only looking for fully clothed ladies in big hats! 'Honestly guv, nothing sinister'. Even today, all these years later, it is not uncommon for some dealers (perhaps with delusions of grandeur?) not even to bother stocking this type of card at all and, on occasion, one is smartly directed to the 50p box where all the dross is kept! Visiting French and continental dealers on the other hand, apparently innately appreciating the finer points of ladies fashion, seem very much more on the ball than us Anglo Saxons and my requests of 'Avez-vous Les Modes?' have often yielded great riches. Similarly, the countless hours spent trawling through literally hundreds of thousands of cards in some large hall or other around the country over the years, could, if you were lucky, prove to be time well spent and add a few more members to my family of Edwardian 'girlfriends'. Those who have spent eons of their lives in the pastime of fishing will have a reasonable concept of what I mean!

Lost in Time

So who were these pretty young fashion models of their day, these timeless beauties, coyly smiling out at us? Well, sad to say, that from amongst all the many cards that I have – apart from the cards of named actresses and stage celebrities – few if any offer the identity of the sitter. Nameless child models were also all the rage and huge numbers of Shirley-Temple-like children were featured.

Sadly, a hundred years on, Father Time has taken his toll and all the models featured in my collection have inevitably made their way to the great photographic studio in the sky, so their names will remain forever lost to us. But for sure, while their names are unknown today, this was their moment in time; their little bit of fame maybe and a way for a pretty girl to spice up her life and make a little extra money.

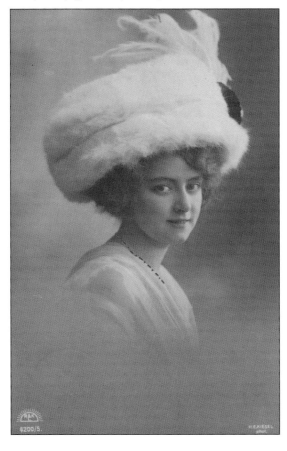

Many of the models appear time and time again in various different get ups and hats and they must have been well recognised in their day as the equivalent of the catwalk 'lovelies' that we see strutting their stuff today or featured in the 'glossies'. But the irony of the whole situation is that whilst these young ladies featured on the postcards looked happy, smiling and elegant, behind this fashion facade lurked the 'killing fields' and the decimation and brutalisation of millions of birds. Like all fashion models, many of them must have worked on various different assignments with postcards being just one aspect of their work. Appearances on sets of playing cards were not unknown and indeed, I did once spot that one of these nameless models in her fancy hat had somehow managed to appear on the label on top of an Edwardian box of Christmas crackers – fame indeed.

Anonymity, as already mentioned, did not strictly apply to all the models however – especially in showbiz circles. Usually mass produced in black and white format,

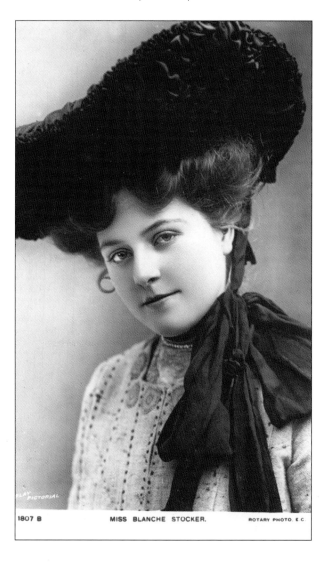

1807 B   MISS BLANCHE STOCKER.   ROTARY PHOTO. E.C.

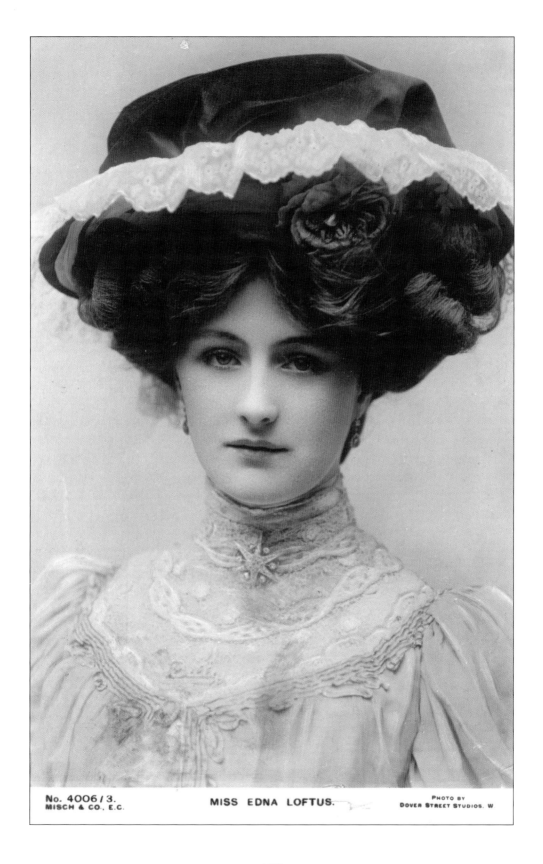

No. 4006/3.
MISCH & CO., E.C.

MISS EDNA LOFTUS.

PHOTO BY
DOVER STREET STUDIOS. W

159

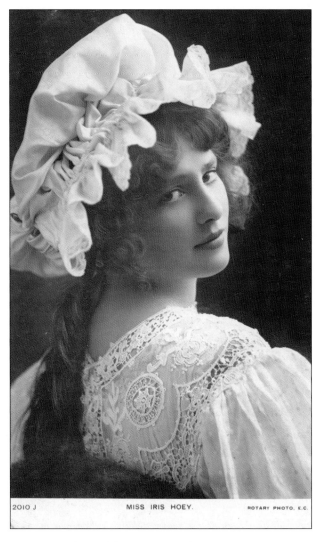

2010 J   MISS IRIS HOEY.   ROTARY PHOTO. E.C.

there were many postcards which promoted numerous actresses of the period across Europe – published by the likes of Bassano, Reutlinger (operating in Paris from 1850 – 1937), Beagles and Davidson Bros. Well known stage, dance and music hall personalities such as Zena and Phyllis Dare, Gabrielle and Ruby Ray, Marie Lohr, Iris Hoey, Kitty Mason, Billie Burke, Mabel Love and those two beauties Gladys Cooper and the delicious Lily Elsie amongst the many, may all be seen smiling at us from under their enormous and outrageous hats. At 2d for black and white and 3d for coloured, the choice was yours. Risqué cards too, especially continental, were readily available and it was not unknown for the Reutlinger company to source its best photographic models from such places as the Folies Bergère, the Comedie Français and the Opéra Bouffe. These 'Actress' cards – invariably carrying the name of the celebrity – were published in great quantities and eagerly sort after by their armies of fans. I did once read somewhere that Gladys Cooper had many linen

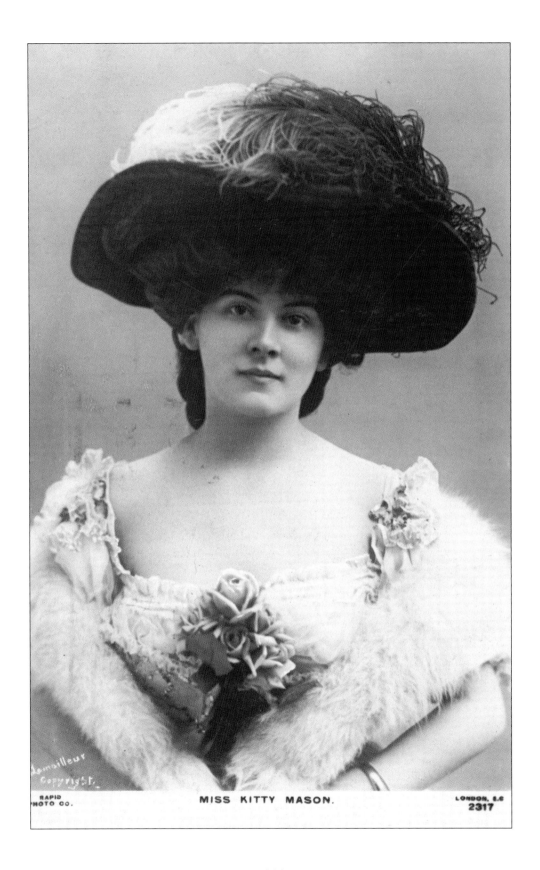

RAPID
PHOTO CO.

MISS KITTY MASON.

LONDON, S.C
2317

baskets crammed full of postcards from her numerous admirers, and it was also reported that there was a period earlier in her career when she and others, (many of whom signed lucrative contracts with the card publishers) were earning significantly more money from being photographed for postcards (frequently sporting large feathered hats) than she was bringing in from acting. The millinery trade must have loved her.

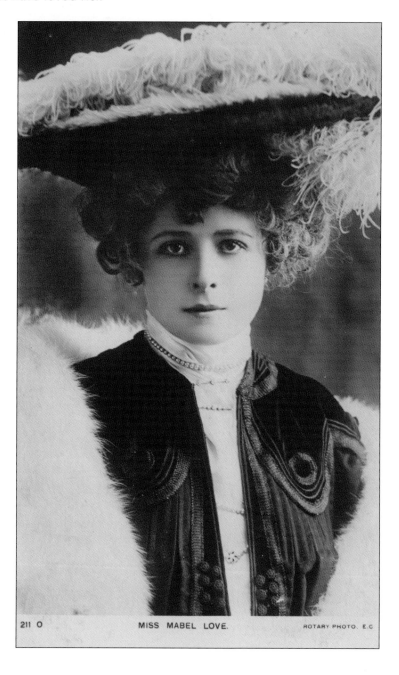

211 O   MISS MABEL LOVE.   ROTARY PHOTO. E.C

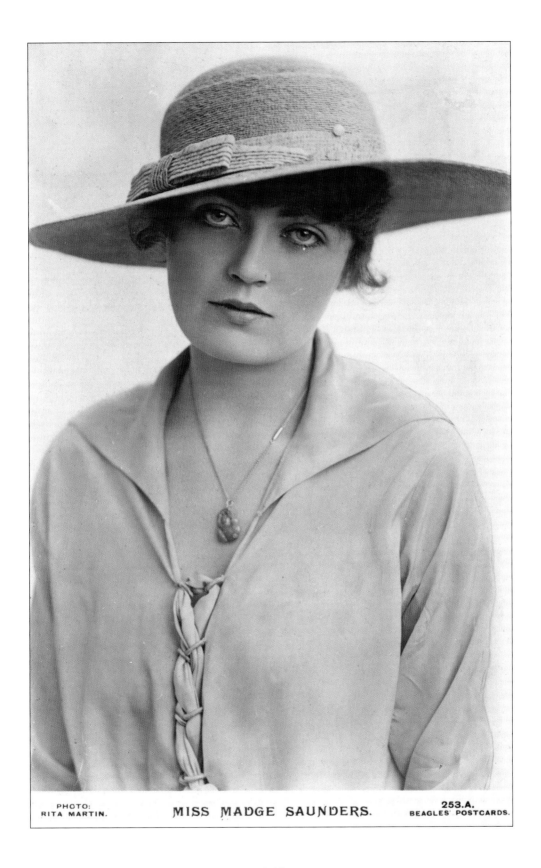

PHOTO:
RITA MARTIN.   MISS MADGE SAUNDERS.   253.A.
BEAGLES' POSTCARDS.

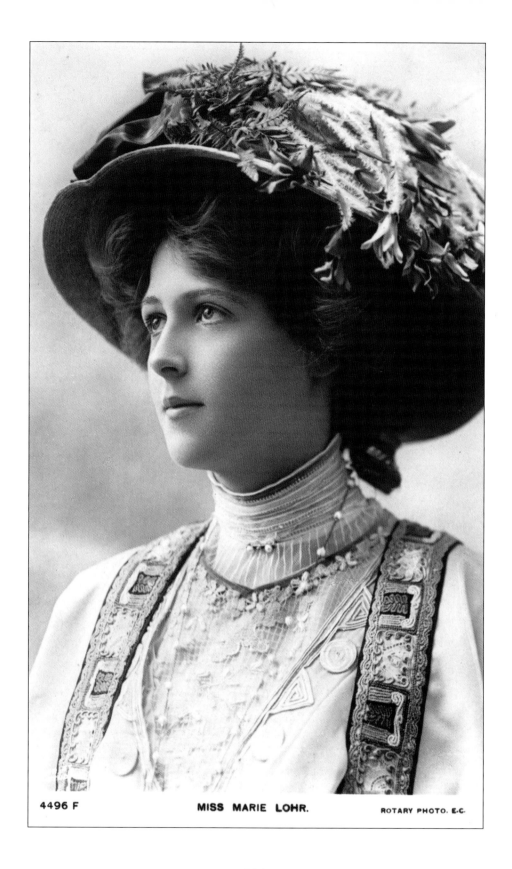

4496 F   MISS MARIE LOHR.   ROTARY PHOTO. E.C.

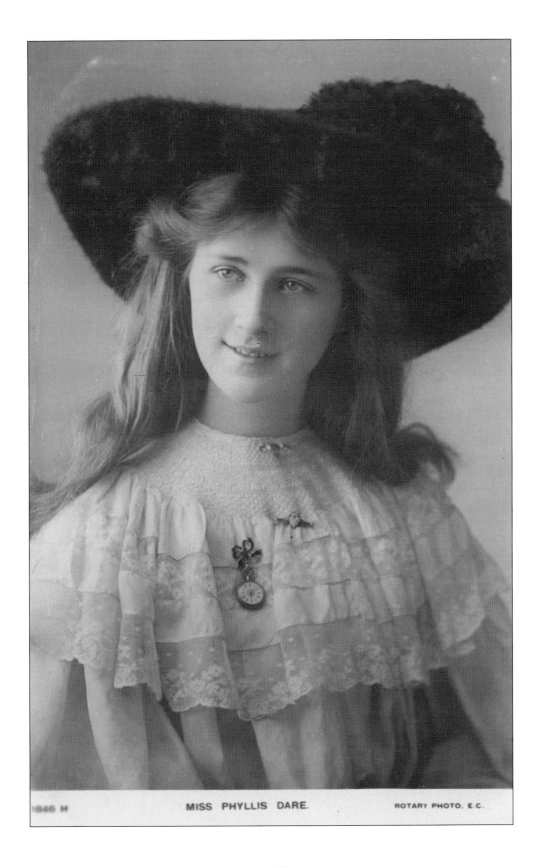

MISS PHYLLIS DARE.

1846 H   ROTARY PHOTO. E.C.

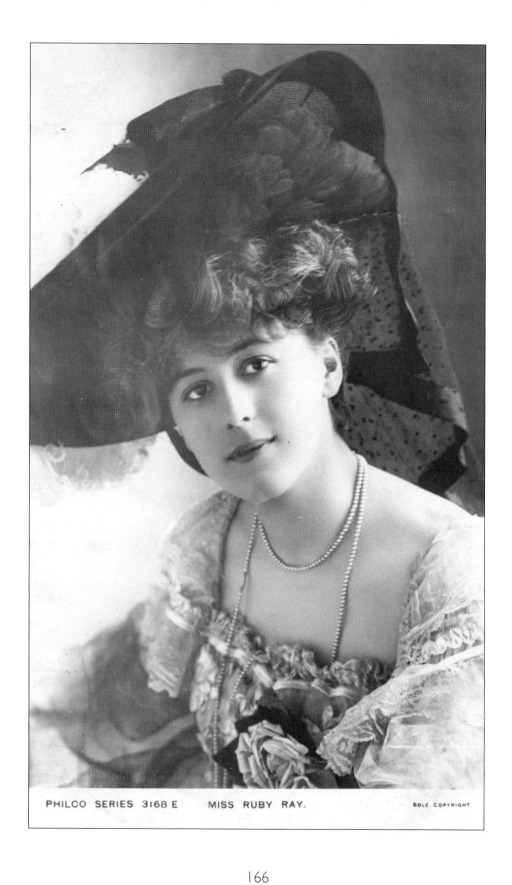

PHILCO SERIES 3168 E   MISS RUBY RAY.   SOLE COPYRIGHT

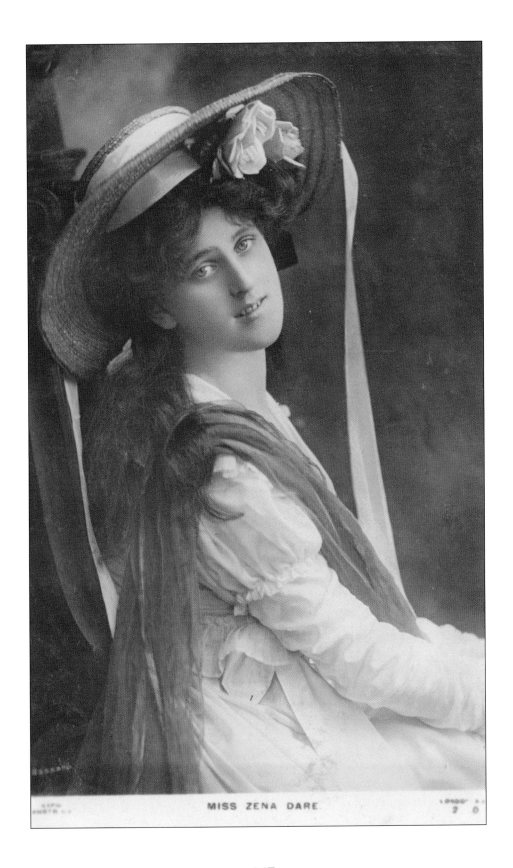

MISS ZENA DARE.

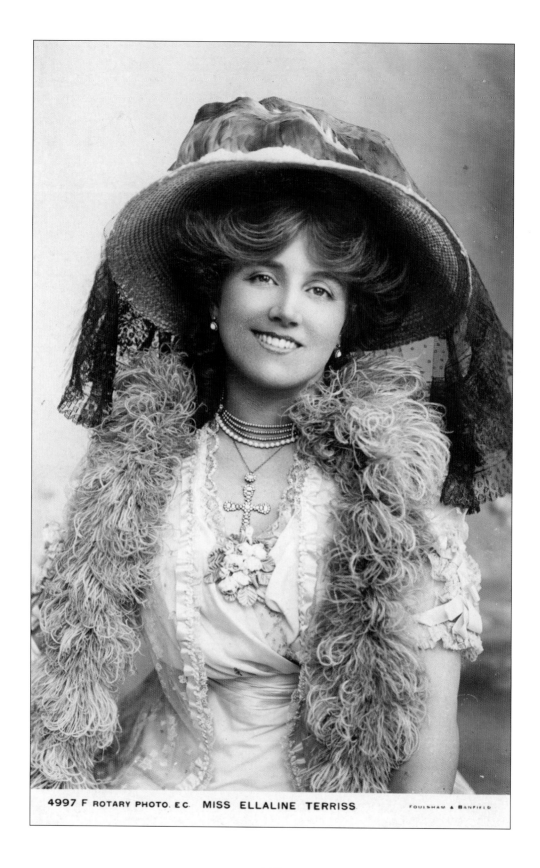

4997 F ROTARY PHOTO. E.C. MISS ELLALINE TERRISS. FOULSHAM & BANFIELD

168

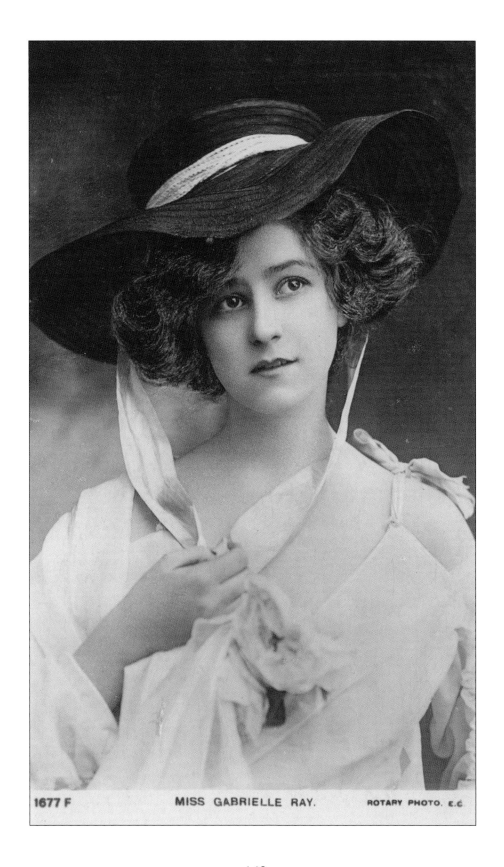

1677 F   MISS GABRIELLE RAY.   ROTARY PHOTO. E.C

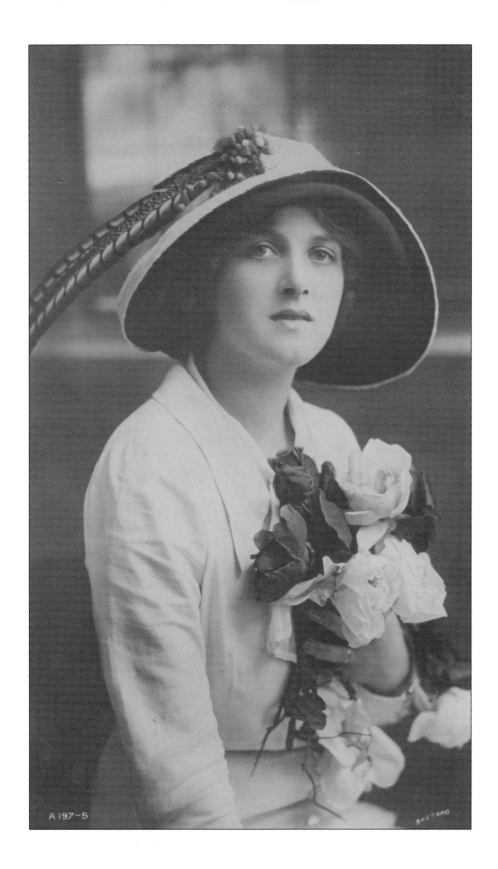

Down with the Hun!

Many of the photographic glamour postcards of the later Edwardian period featuring feather-covered hats were listed as being 'Printed in Prussia' (or Germany and sometimes Saxony). But sadly, the storm clouds of conflict were inexorably gathering and, with ill feeling in both Britain and Germany on the rise, it is not uncommon to see on the back of some cards that the country of origin has been obliterated or scratched out – probably by the retailer on account of the growing ill-feeling towards the German people leading up to and including the war period. From a retailing and sales point of view, the public were surely not going to patronise establishments offering postcards printed in the enemy's homeland however pretty the young lady on the front! Nevertheless, wartime or not, the quality of printing coming out of this region was invariably and by tradition, extremely good.

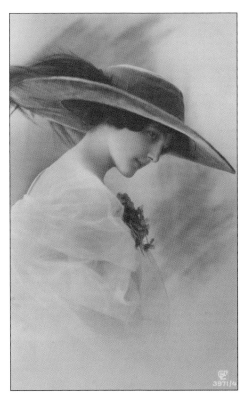

Keeping the Presses Rolling

Such was their popularity – covering, as we have said, a huge range of subjects, that the postcard publishers of the period must have had an absolute field day and names which particularly stood out as producing real quality photo 'Glamour' images were: The Carlton Publishing Company, Rotary Photo, Raphael Tuck, Schwerdleger & Company, Ettlingers and Alfred Stiebel to name but a few. It is estimated that by the early 1900s, the publishers were producing around 50,000 postcards per day and it was said that the national UK population of 37 million at that time was mailing 600 million postcards annually! By 1910, that figure had risen by an astonishing fifty per cent, to the extent that a large industry arose to supply whole ranges of beautifully decorated albums to house people's collections. Even today, though often in a somewhat 'tatty' condition, these albums still regularly turn up at antique fairs and auctions.

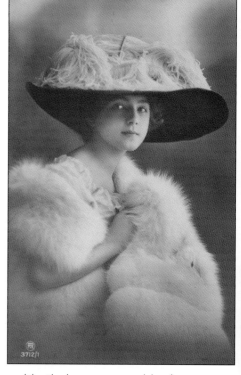

Conversely, as with the models, the actual photographers never seem to get a mention with the notable exception of one well known 'snapper' by the name of H E KIESEL – who always seems to have his name on the front of any postcards featuring his work. He was undoubtedly very accomplished and constantly produced a variety of attractive poses – invariably getting the best from his sitters. There were also many artists who came up with their own graphic (as opposed to photographic) interpretations of these young ladies in their hats and the names of C.W. Barber, Lawrence Miller and E.H. Kiefer quite frequently appear.

Gilding the Lily

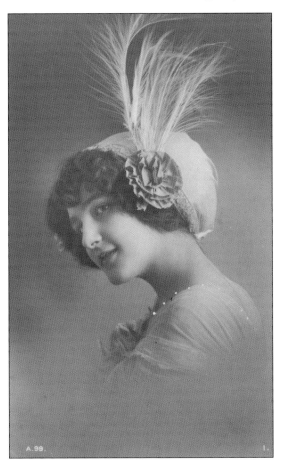

s previously mentioned, the 'Glamour' cards themselves were nearly always produced in sets of six different poses of the same young lady model, as a basic matt sepia-toned (or plain black and white) print which then had the colours for the flesh tones, hats and dresses etc. added in the publisher's own colouring factories or by female home workers and/or outworkers. Sometimes, little bits of real feathers, slivers of material or in some cases glitter were stuck to the face of the cards to create a sort of 3D or decorative effect and it is often possible to find little hand embossed dots forming a part of the presentation.

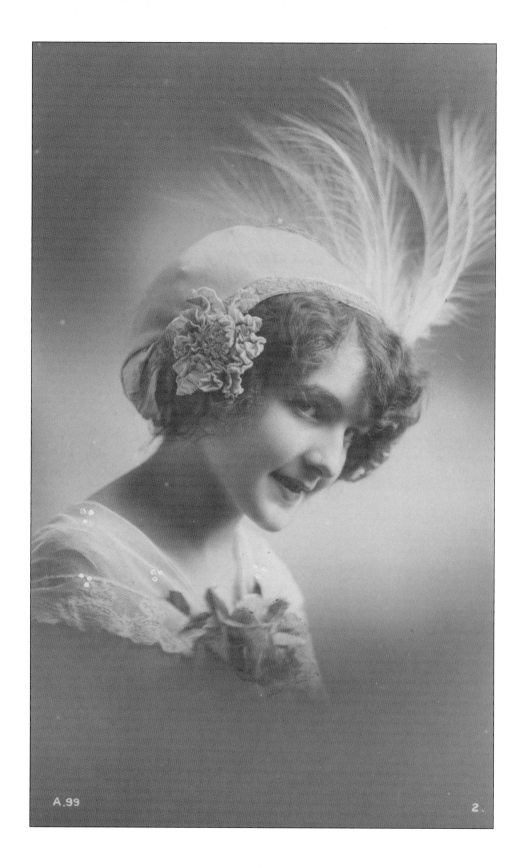

A.99

2.

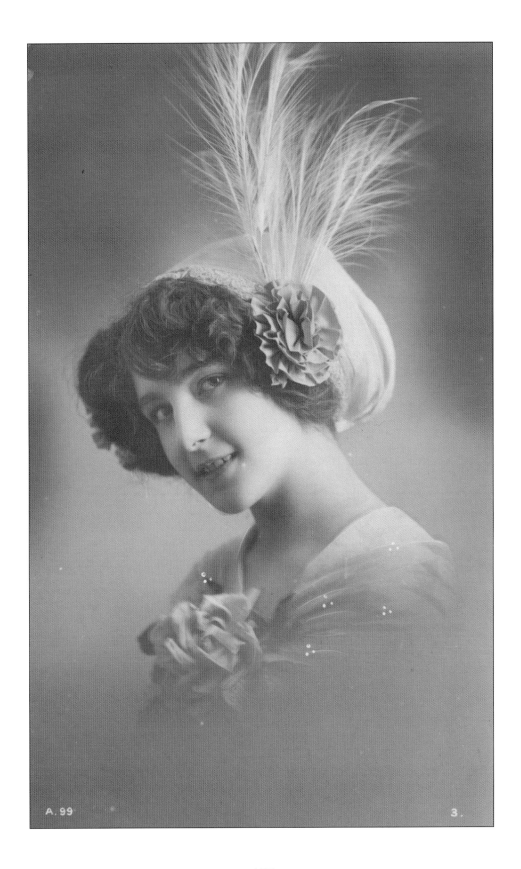

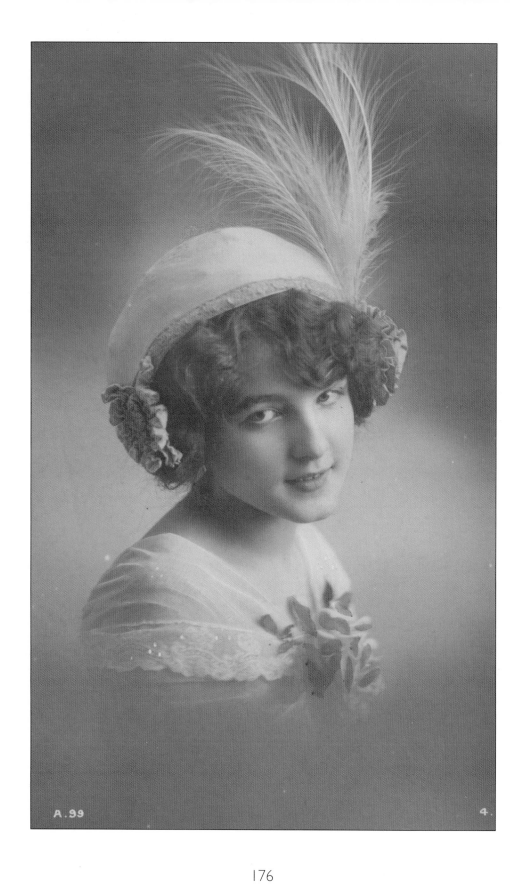

A.99   4.

Colour photography of a reasonable standard had not yet really come into play (which it finally did in the mid 1930s) and the girls would colour the cards by hand with oil based inks, photo tints or paints which at times caused illness because the ladies, as they worked, would often lick their brushes to get a better point. These complete sets which are pretty hard to find these days, would have a basic code number at the bottom left or right with a suffix number added at the end. You would therefore have a simple coding system something along the lines of – 33445/1, 33445/2, and so on up to /6. Colouring standards varied greatly with the more skilled colourists doing a great job – producing accurate and tasteful work, while the less accomplished often spoiled the end result with pretty inferior, and at times slap-dash, standards. Although I have never been able to find any images of these ladies at work, one can perhaps imagine the factory work benches or for outworkers, dining tables and maybe even the floors of the colourists' homes being strewn with cards as each individual colour was added and put aside to dry. I've yet to discover what was the going rate to colour, say, a dozen or a gross of cards but it certainly can't have been that much.

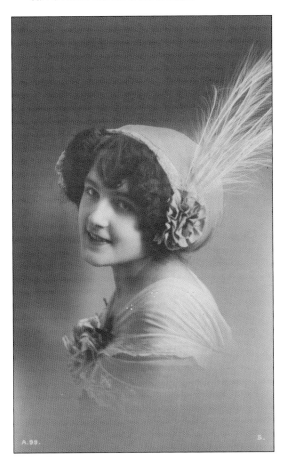 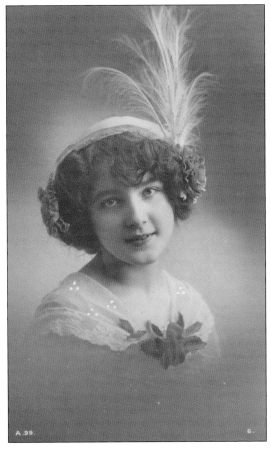

From the Trenches

From my own large collection of 'Hat' cards, people often ask me which is my favourite and, on the face of it, you might think that to be a difficult choice. But no. In my case it is a very easy one to answer. My absolute favourite and most treasured card is not the most expensive and certainly not the most skilfully coloured.

The image which I like best of all is that of a charming young lady, not in a feather covered hat but in a frilly lace 'milk maid' style bonnet, which cost me just a mere forty pence many years ago and which was sent by a humble First World War soldier signing himself only as Brian – probably serving in the trenches. I am advised by the Imperial War Museum that from time to time, the troops were granted a certain amount of time off from the carnage to 'relax' (if that were possible) behind the lines and it is a fair guess that Brian probably purchased this card in one of the nearby towns or villages that somehow had remained standing or, from whatever was the equivalent of the NAAFI in those days. His message was just one of the estimated 12.5 million that were being sent home by soldiers each week. All correspondence was supposedly vetted and he was duty bound in what he wrote to say nothing that would help the enemy.

Addressed to his beloved sister, a Miss J.W. Porter at 'Mountlands', Upper Bridge St. in Redhill, Surrey with the still barely visible stamps of 'Official Censor' and 'Field Post Office', the reverse of the card simply reads:

'On Active Service – Wednesday morning December 13th 1916.'

He writes:

We had quite a heavy fall of snow today but most of it has disappeared already. Thought you might like this card, which struck me as being very pretty. You will be glad to hear that the stoppage of leave was only temporary as it has started again this morning. Have got over guard alright – with only the addition of a slight cold.

Much love to all from your affectionate brother – Brian.

Poignant and yet so evocative of those terrible times when huge numbers of loved ones failed to return. Winter in the trenches in December 1916 must have been an utter nightmare – a truly daunting prospect even for the most hardy of souls! Of around the 720,000 British soldiers that are said to have perished, did Brian manage to survive? Very possibly not, and I often wonder if he ever made it back home again to stroll arm in arm with his beloved sister 'J' in her big feathered hat.

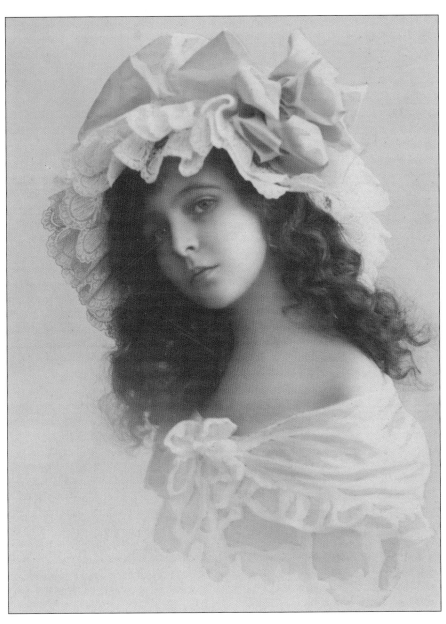

Another amazing hat in 'Milkmaid' style – featured on a poignant postcard sent in 1916 from somewhere in the First World War battlefields of France by a soldier named Brian to his sister 'J' in Surrey. (See what he wrote on Page 180)

Hope for the Birds!

Well, traditionalist I may be, perhaps even an overly incurable romantic – use any tag you like but whatever, nobody can deny that these evocative period postcards from their short window in history are a wonderful source of reference for today's students of the fashion trends of that bygone era when these stunning, feather adorned hats were very much a 'must have' accessory for the elegant young ladies of the day.

Although they are indeed long gone, such is the crazy world we live in today that, coupled with the creativity of modern day fashion gurus, it's not beyond the realms of possibility that one day we just may see a designer or two promoting the mass return of these astonishing feathered creations. Impossible? You would almost certainly think so but, with the world being such a mad place where seemingly, anything goes, I would never bet against it. Fortunately, for the present at least, our feathered friends can rest more easily in knowing that today's more enlightened conservationists and protection lobbies around the world – especially the RSPB in the UK and the National Audubon Society in America – wielding much greater clout than in those earlier days, would have a very great deal to say about that. Opposition would be fierce for sure – and rightly so.

And so in summary, we've looked at the amazing ladies' hat fashions of the Edwardian period and we've looked at the depths to which at least some of the human race sank in its brutal treatment of the avian population – purely in pursuit of money and in satisfying the fashion trends of the day. Thankfully, there were those enlightened folk around at the time who tried their best to do something about it and sowed the seeds of change.

For my part, while appreciating that we cannot change what has happened in the past, I'm firmly on the side of the birds and I'll stick to my postcards. But nonetheless, I hope you have enjoyed meeting just a few of my Edwardian 'girlfriends', their youthful faces captured forever in time, in their amazing feathered creations. Long gone they may be, but thanks to the postcards of the day, their images live on.

Gosh Granny, 'Where Did You Get That Hat?'

Appendix 1

Hats, Fashion and Textiles Around the World

Did they really used to dress like that? A question often asked. Fashion in all its many forms and from whatever period of history provides an ongoing fascination for millions of people around the planet. Indeed, we can only guess at the overall size of the world's fashion industry today in all its forms and the contribution it brings to the international economy. For the huge number of people around the globe with an interest in period millinery, fashion in general and textiles, the following list offers details of some of the more notable fashion museums, collections and archives in the United Kingdom, North America, mainland Europe and around the world. These venues offer much to interest both locals and visitors alike and I am greatly indebted to the knowledgeable Anne Bissonnette Phd – Curator, Clothing and Textile Collection, University of Alberta, Canada for her generous input and expertise in providing this information.

United Kingdom:
Victoria & Albert Museum, London. www.vam.ac.uk
Also view – collections.vam.ac.uk
Museum of London. www.museumoflondon.org.uk
Wardown Park Museum. www.wardownparkmuseum.com
Stockport Hat Works Museum. www.stockport.gov.uk/hatworks
The Fashion Museum, Bath. www.museumofcostume.co.uk
Norwich Castle Study Centre.
www.museums.norfolk.gov.uk

North America:
The Hat Museum, Portland, Oregon. www.thehatmuseum.com
Fashion Institute of Technology, New York. www.fitnyc.edu
Philadelphia Museum of Art. www.philamuseum.org
Los Angeles County Museum of Art. www.lacma.org
Museum of Fine Arts, Boston. www.mfa.org

Museum of Fine Arts, Houston. www.mfah.org
Ohio State University Costume Collection. www.costume.osu.edu
University of Alberta Clothing & Textile Collection. www.ualberta.ca
Costume Museum of Canada. www.costumemuseum.com
Museum of Costume & Textile of Quebec. www.mctq.org
Royal Alberta Museum. www.royalalbertamuseum.ca
Royal Ontario Museum. www.rom.on.ca
Phoenix Art Museum, Costume Department. www.phxart.org
Texas Fashion Collection. www.tfc.unt.edu
Textile Museum (Washinton DC). www.textilemuseum.org
The Valentine Museum, Costumes and Textiles. www.richmondhistorycenter.com
de Young Museum, Textile Arts Collection. www.deyoung.famsf.org
Kent State University Museum. www.kent.edu
FIDM Museum. www.fidmmuseum.org
Museum of Art, Rhode Island School of Design. Costume/Textiles. www.ridsmuseum.org
Museum of the City of New York. Fashion, Costumes and Textiles.
   www.collections.mcny.org-United States
Costume Institute at the Metropolitan Museum of Art, New York.
   www.metmuseum.org

Europe:
Musée des Arts Décoratifs. www.lesartsdecoratifs.fr
Espace Mode Mediterranée. www.m-mmm.fr
Musée de la Mode de la Ville de Paris, Paris Galliera. www.museums-of-paris.com
Musée de L'impression sur Etoffes,Mulhouse. www.musee-impression.com
Mode Museum, Antwerp. www.momu.be
German Historical Museum. Textiles and Clothes Department. www.dhm.de

International:
The Costume Museum of Japan. www.fashionmuseum.or.jp
Kyoto Costume Institute. www.kci.or.jp
The C.P. Nel Museum, Oudtshoorn, Western Cape Province, South Africa.
   www.cpnelmuseum.co.za

Professional Organisations:
Costume Society of America. www.costumesocietyamerica.com
Costume Society of Great Britain. www.costumesociety.org.uk
International Council of Museums. www.icom.museum
International Textiles and Apparel Association. www.itaaonline.org
The Textile Society (UK). www.textilesociety.org.uk
The Textile Society of America. www.textilesociety.org

Appendix 2

A Century of Bird Protection

I n the enduring words of one time Director of the New York Zoological Park – William Temple Hornaday, the American zoologist and naturalist who wrote in his 1913 book – *Our Vanishing Wildlife*:

We are weary of witnessing the greed, selfishness and cruelty of 'civilised' man toward the wild creatures of the earth. We are sick of the slaughter and pictures of carnage. It is time for sweeping reformation and that is precisely what we now demand.

With those sentiments to the fore and by way of conclusion, I am pleased to include the following direct contributions from both the RSPB here in the UK and the National Audubon Society of America which, in their own words, give the reader a brief insight into the early years of these organisations and reminds us all that both we and the birds are lucky to have them. Without them, the world would be a poorer place and with the sentiments of Hornaday in mind, we should be enduringly grateful for their work.

THE AUDUBON SOCIETY OF AMERICA

Just in Time

A little over 100 years ago, the conservation movement took flight… and not a minute too soon. By 1900, Americans' belief that our continent's wildlife was inexhaustible, had led to serious consequences. Bison no longer roamed the Great Plains, and Passenger Pigeons that had once darkened the skies for miles as they passed overhead – had been exterminated. Many other species were on the brink. Overhunting and habitat destruction were key factors. But in the case of birds something else was also at work. A new fashion had swept the nation — bird hats were all the rage.

One day while walking in Manhattan, Frank Chapman — publisher of *Bird Lore* magazine — counted: 542 people wearing hats adorned with either entire birds or their plumage — representing a total of forty-two bird species. Egrets, in particular, were so highly prized that their feathers were worth twice their weight in gold. No wonder that plume hunters were slaughtering them. But through the bold efforts of some farsighted Americans, these magnificent creatures and many more were saved ... just in time. It was these men and women who founded one of America's longest-lived and most successful conservation organizations — the National Audubon Society.

The story of Audubon begins a few years earlier, in 1886 when New York publisher, George Bird Grinnell, invited readers of his *Forest & Stream* magazine to sign a pledge that they would not harm birds. He named this eager group the Audubon Society for the Protection of Birds, named after the famed bird and wildlife artist, John James Audubon. But response was so great he couldn't keep up and reluctantly had to fold the organization. A decade later, Harriet Hemenway used her home in Boston as the gathering spot for friends who vowed to stop the continued destruction of wildlife. These women started a grassroots movement that quickly became the Massachusetts Audubon Society.

From there, Audubon Societies sprang up across the country. Finally, on 5 January 1905 in New York City, leaders from thirty-one state organizations formed the National Association of Audubon Societies for the Protection of Wild Birds and Animals, later to be named the National Audubon Society. Prominent ornithologist William Dutcher served as its first president.

A Deadly Battle

Early bird conservation meant waging battles on two fronts. On one, influential citizens persuaded their friends not to create demand for bird plumes ... on the supply front, the struggle turned deadly. In Florida — the epicenter of the plumage trade — Audubon hired wardens to protect vital bird nesting sites. Guy Bradley was one of these wardens. He himself had been a plume hunter, but had come to believe the decimation had to stop. On confronting a poacher he knew, Bradley was shot and killed, and left to drift in his boat. Over the next three years, two more Audubon wardens would be shot and killed in the line of duty. Their deaths became the rallying cry for conservationists across the country.

Friends in High Places

One of them was President Theodore Roosevelt. An ardent conservationist and ornithologist, Roosevelt understood that natural areas and wildlife were in serious danger unless protected. And so he created the nation's first wildlife refuge – Florida's Pelican Island – in 1903, followed by five of our National Parks, fifty-one Bird Preserves and 150 National Forests. Roosevelt became known fittingly as the 'conservation President'. He also became an Honorary Vice President of the Audubon Society, which was in turn, motivated by his passion, and his pragmatism.

Audubon's Mission
'To conserve and restore natural ecosystems. Focusing on birds, other wildlife and their habitats for the benefit of humanity and the earth's biological diversity.'

THE ROYAL SOCIETY FOR THE PROTECTION OF BIRDS

United Kingdom
On a wing and a prayer...
The RSPB was formed to counter the barbarous trade in plumes for women's hats, a fashion responsible for the destruction of many thousands of egrets, birds of paradise and other species whose plumes had become fashionable in the late Victorian era.

There had already been concern earlier in the century about the wholesale destruction of such native birds as great crested grebes and kittiwakes for their plumage, leading to such early legislation as the Sea Birds Preservation Act of 1869 and the Wild Birds Protection Act of 1880, but the trigger which led to the foundation of the Society for the Protection of Birds in 1889 was the continued wearing of ever more exotic plumes.

In its earliest days the Society consisted entirely of women who were moved by the emotional appeal of the plight of young birds left to starve in the nest after their parents had been shot for their plumes. Ironically, some of the Society's staunchest supporters were those from the upper classes who would have been the most lightly to have worn feathers.

The rules of the Society were very simple and a number of influential figures, including the leading ornithologist of the day, Professor Alfred Newton lent their support to the cause, which gained widespread publicity and popularity, leading to a rapid growth in the Society's membership and a widening of its aims.

Indeed the young Society was so successful that it was granted its Royal Charter in 1904, just fifteen years after being founded.

The RSPB Today

The RSPB speaks out for birds and wildlife, tackling the problems that threaten our environment.

We are the largest wildlife conservation organisation in Europe with over one million members. Wildlife and the environment face many threats. Our work is focused on the species and habitats that are in the greatest danger.

Our work is driven by the passionate belief that:

- Birds and wildlife enrich people's lives.
- The health of bird populations is indicative of the health of the planet, on which the future of the human race depends.
- We all have a responsibility to protect wildlife.

We have more than one million members, over 18,000 volunteers, 1,300 staff, more than 200 nature reserves, nine regional offices, a UK headquarters, three national offices... and one vision – to work for a better environment rich in birds and wildlife.

The RSPB speaks out for birds and wildlife, tackling the problems that threaten our environment. Nature is amazing – help us keep it that way.

BIRDLIFE INTERNATIONAL

The world's largest civil society Partnership for nature.

In the darkest days of the later Victorian and subsequent Edwardian periods, the carnage visited upon the world's bird populations, simply to garner their feathers for the international fashion industry, was nothing short of nightmare proportions. Happily, things, in the early twenty-first century have fortunately moved on for the better.

Today, as the world's leading global, non-profit making conservation partnership, BirdLife International has more than 13 million members and supporters. This comprises some 2.77 million actual members and a further 10.8 million non member supporters. BirdLife Partner organisations work with over 7,000 local groups including 2,750 Important Bird and Biodiversity Areas including 2.7 million children.

At the start of 2015, BirdLife Partners manage or own 1553 protected areas covering 4.3 million hectares globally of natural areas and employs over 7,000 staff with a combined budget of $589 million. Working with many local communities, the organisation has been described as providing very cost effective action and 'the best bang for buck in the conservation world' with its work on bird conservation in which over 10,000 species are recognised.

The world's oldest truly international conservation organisation

Post First World War, Bird Life's mission 'Was not different from what we have been doing before – namely to work for the conservation of the world's biological diversity and the sustainability of human use of natural resources by focusing on a life-form group which, throughout the history of conservation, has shown itself to be of special importance in recognising and addressing problems affecting our living environment'.

The internationalisation of conservation activities in the form of organisations is essentially a post First World War development. The first international initiatives were taken in North America during the first decade of the twentieth century and in 1910, other attempts were made in Europe; but it was not before 1922 that the first truly international conservation organisation – the international Council for Bird preservation (ICBP) was created.

In May 1928, the ICBP held its first formal conference in Geneva, Switzerland. Resolutions were passed for 'unofficial action' on the creation of bird sanctuaries and the collection of large numbers of the eggs of rare species – ('generally objectionable and unworthy of a good naturalist'). To take into account the diverse legislation and customs of different countries, the Committee felt the best chance of securing international agreement would be to confine its recommendations for official action to two definite proposals. One called for a 'closed season' on the shooting and trapping of birds on their spring migration and while breeding and the other for an international convention on oil pollution, 'which should take into consideration the great loss of birds from this cause'.

Another concern was the mass destruction of birds of prey: not only were these birds not protected but many national and state governments offered bounties which resulted in the slaughter of tens of thousands of hawks and owls every year. The ICBP national sections set out to lobby their governments and raise awareness of the importance of raptors in the 'balance of nature' and as rodent controllers. Slowly, protection was introduced across Europe, though in some Mediterranean countries it was (and in a few cases still is) not enforced.

Therefore, with the nature of mankind being what it is, the job will probably never be totally complete but wonderful strides have been made since those sombre days of the Victorian and Edwardian periods. And for those who may be interested in contributing to the protection and enhancement of the world's wildlife in the years to come, more information may be found on – **www.birdlife.org**

Appendix 3

Museum, Fashion Archives and Societies

Norwich Castle Study Centre
Costume & Textiles Archive

The dedicated follower of fashion will find the Costume and Textile archive – part of the Norwich Castle Study Centre – located centrally in the fine City of Norwich, England; one not to miss. In using the Study Centre, you will be able to focus on specific collections and select the objects and areas you wish to see in support of your area of interest.

Situated in the old Shirehall and attached to the old law court, this excellent, relaxed and comprehensive facility containing over 27,000 items reflects changing fashions, styles and technology in the varied clothing, accessories and textiles of all sexes and ages across the eighteenth, nineteenth and twentieth centuries. From the vast range of material available, of particular interest is the largest collection of Norwich Shawls in the country. For those with a particular interest in Edwardian hat fashions, one may journey back in time and view many examples of fashion and women's magazines, craft magazines and journals, trade and exhibition catalogues and specialist costume and textile society publications together with fashion plates and photographs dating back to the mid-nineteenth century.

You may examine your chosen items of interest in the peace and tranquility of one of the dedicated study rooms. Here, objects and material from the collections are brought to you by friendly and well-informed staff who are pleased to assist visitors with their specialist knowledge.

Open to the public by pre-booked appointment only.

To discuss your requirements in advance,
Email : museums@norfolk.gov.uk
www.museums.norfolk.gov.uk

The Hat Museum
Portland, Oregon, USA

The Hat Museum (also known as The National Hat Museum) is an exhibit of over 1,300 hats – carefully chosen from among the most characteristic styles of past eras, providing a wide-ranging historical perspective on what has always been THE essential accessory. This is a full spectrum museum that exhibits men's and women's hats together with children's, military, novelty, hats worn in Hollywood movies and features international hats from over fifty countries.

The women's hats date back to 1837 and the men's to 1850. Featured are Victorian hats, Edwardian, flapper cloche hats and examples from all decades up to the present day. Men's examples include tricorn, top, Homburg, bowler, fedora, trilby, fez, cowboy and many military examples. It also houses twenty-three brand name designer hats in the collection. Period accessories such as purses, gloves, parasols and eyeglasses are also incorporated into the hat displays.

The Hat Museum, regularly featured in the media, has offered tours since 1990, is listed on the National Historic Registry and is housed in the historic Ladd-Reingold House just a few minutes by car from downtown Portland, Oregon.

One point to remember is that the museum is not open to the general public. Tours (by reservation only) are offered to costumiers, fashion and history academics and millinery students. Those interested in visiting should check directly with the museum in advance. The Hat Museum also offers vintage hats for sale.

As far as North America is concerned and for visitors from around the globe, this attraction is certainly well worth a visit.

www.thehatmuseum.com
www.thehatmuseum.etsy.com

The American Hatpin Society

The American Hatpin Society is an international club of collectors of vintage hatpins and holders (1890-1920). Members enjoy a colourful and informative newsletter and quarterly luncheon-meetings featuring various speakers, hatpins and holders.

Founded in May 1989 by a group of enthusiastic hatpin and hatpin holder collectors, the purpose of the society is to provide information about the history and value of hatpins and hatpin holders.

The Society accepts membership from all over the world and has special arrangements for members in the USA.

Contact: American Hatpin Society President – Jodi Lenocker
P.O.Box 2672 Lake Arrowhead, CA 92352
www.americanhatpinsociety.com

The CP Nel Museum – Oudtshoorn
Western Cape Province, South Africa

For anyone with even a passing interest in Edwardian fashion and, by association, the feather industry of that period, a visit to the town of Oudtshoorn in South Africa, for over one hundred years the worldwide centre of the ostrich feather industry, is a must. Similarly, whilst there, a trip to the C.P. Nel Museum will tell you all you need to know about the subject and, coupled with the beautiful surrounding Western Cape Province countryside, will make any visit well worthwhile.

The Museum, which was declared a National Monument in 1981, has a whole section devoted to the ostrich feather industry and owes its origins to the private collection of the late Colonel Charles Paul Nel – a successful businessman and collector who entrusted his collection to the Museum's Board of Trustees shortly before he died in 1951. He must surely be remembered with gratitude for having the foresight to put together what is certainly a unique record of the industry.

Ostrich feather farming brought unparalleled prosperity to the Klein Karoo during the late nineteenth century and a legacy from this economic boom is the distinctive sandstone architecture, which includes a number of the so-called 'Ostrich Feather Palaces'. Today two of these impressive buildings form part of the C.P. Nel Museum complex in Baron van Reede Street. **www.cpnelmuseum.co.za**

This Cultural History Museum of Oudtshoorn and the Little Karoo region, is a declared national monument and houses exhibitions showcasing the fascinating story of the ostrich feather industry.

3 Baron van Reede St. T: +27 (0)44 272 7306 F: +27 (0)86 553 9226
Email: cpnelmanager@mweb.co.za Website: www.cpnelmuseum.co.za
Postal Address: PO Box 453 Oudtshoorn 6620 South Africa
Hours: Monday-Friday from 08:00 to 17:00
Saturday from 09:00 to 13:00

Linley Sambourne House
18 Stafford Terrace
London, England

As may be seen on page ? Edward Linley Sambourne was the celebrated *Punch* cartoonist, illustrator and photographer. Many of his 'secret' photographic fashion images featuring lovely young Edwardian ladies from the early years of the twentieth century in their super-sized hats, (a selection of which are featured in this book) may be viewed, by appointment, at 18 Stafford Terrace (Linley Sambourne House) in Kensington in London. If fashion holds an interest for you, particularly from the reign of Edward VII then why not make time to visit this superb photographic archive of Sambourne's images, which really should not be missed!
www.rbkc.gov.uk/museum

Author Details

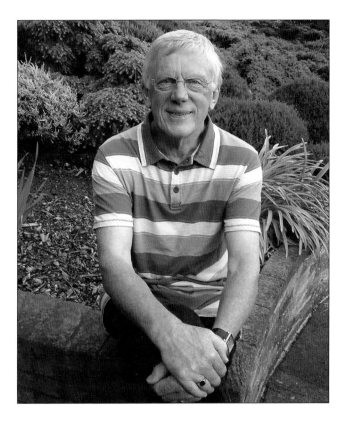

Aged 75 and born in Tetbury, Gloucestershire, England, July 1941.

Educated at the City of Norwich Grammar School from 1952 to 1957.

Amongst the positions I have held, were twenty-three years with the confectionery manufacturer, John Mackintosh (subsequently Rowntree Mackintosh) based in Norwich, twelve of which, as UK Design Studio Manager, involving graphic design, conceptual packaging development and print for the company products.

I also worked for several years as a Freelance Design Consultant.
I spent six years (1986–1992) as Marketing Services Manager with the Tom Smith Christmas Cracker company, when it was based in Norwich.

I am the world's only Christmas Cracker historian and collector for nearly forty years, of beautiful hand-tinted, early twentieth century Photographic Glamour postcards, and I am also the owner of the Kathleen Kimpton Victorian Photographic Archive.

I decided to write my first book on Tom Smith and the History of the Christmas Cracker in 2000, when I discovered that, apart from the 'potted' history which I had produced when working for Tom Smith's in the late 1980's, an in depth book on the subject had never been undertaken before.

I have given lectures and written and contributed widely on the subject of Christmas Crackers, in the press and in the media, and in 2009 took part in the BBC's *Victorian Farm* programme, to talk about crackers and their history. I have also appeared on the Russian TV (Channel 1), Deutsche Welle – German TV, BBC Breakfast, Mustard TV in Norfolk and various local radio stations around the UK to talk on Cracker history and traditions.